Nathalie Lötscher Petrus

Anaemia Management in dialysis patients in Switzerland
"AIMS"

Nathalie Lötscher Petrus

Anaemia Management in dialysis patients in Switzerland "AIMS"

Assessing the quality of anaemia control and the relevance of individualized anaemia management in dialysis patients

Südwestdeutscher Verlag für Hochschulschriften

Impressum/Imprint (nur für Deutschland/ only for Germany)
Bibliografische Information der Deutschen Nationalbibliothek: Die Deutsche Nationalbibliothek verzeichnet diese Publikation in der Deutschen Nationalbibliografie; detaillierte bibliografische Daten sind im Internet über http://dnb.d-nb.de abrufbar.
Alle in diesem Buch genannten Marken und Produktnamen unterliegen warenzeichen-, marken- oder patentrechtlichem Schutz bzw. sind Warenzeichen oder eingetragene Warenzeichen der jeweiligen Inhaber. Die Wiedergabe von Marken, Produktnamen, Gebrauchsnamen, Handelsnamen, Warenbezeichnungen u.s.w. in diesem Werk berechtigt auch ohne besondere Kennzeichnung nicht zu der Annahme, dass solche Namen im Sinne der Warenzeichen- und Markenschutzgesetzgebung als frei zu betrachten wären und daher von jedermann benutzt werden dürften.

Verlag: Südwestdeutscher Verlag für Hochschulschriften Aktiengesellschaft & Co. KG
Dudweiler Landstr. 99, 66123 Saarbrücken, Deutschland
Telefon +49 681 37 20 271-1, Telefax +49 681 37 20 271-0, Email: info@svh-verlag.de
Zugl.: Basel, phil.-nat., 2005

Herstellung in Deutschland:
Schaltungsdienst Lange o.H.G., Berlin
Books on Demand GmbH, Norderstedt
Reha GmbH, Saarbrücken
Amazon Distribution GmbH, Leipzig
ISBN: 978-3-8381-1090-5

Imprint (only for USA, GB)
Bibliographic information published by the Deutsche Nationalbibliothek: The Deutsche Nationalbibliothek lists this publication in the Deutsche Nationalbibliografie; detailed bibliographic data are available in the Internet at http://dnb.d-nb.de.
Any brand names and product names mentioned in this book are subject to trademark, brand or patent protection and are trademarks or registered trademarks of their respective holders. The use of brand names, product names, common names, trade names, product descriptions etc. even without a particular marking in this works is in no way to be construed to mean that such names may be regarded as unrestricted in respect of trademark and brand protection legislation and could thus be used by anyone.

Publisher:
Südwestdeutscher Verlag für Hochschulschriften Aktiengesellschaft & Co. KG
Dudweiler Landstr. 99, 66123 Saarbrücken, Germany
Phone +49 681 37 20 271-1, Fax +49 681 37 20 271-0, Email: info@svh-verlag.de

Copyright © 2009 by the author and Südwestdeutscher Verlag für Hochschulschriften Aktiengesellschaft & Co. KG and licensors
All rights reserved. Saarbrücken 2009

Printed in the U.S.A.
Printed in the U.K. by (see last page)
ISBN: 978-3-8381-1090-5

*A*naem*I*a *M*anagement in dialysis patients in *S*witzerland "AIMS"

INAUGURALDISSERTATION

zur

Erlangung der Würde eines Doktors der Philosophie

vorgelegt der

Philosophisch-Naturwissenschaftlichen Fakultät der

Universität Basel

von

Nathalie G. Lötscher

aus Oberems (VS)

Basel 2005

Genehmigt von der Philosophisch-Naturwissenschaftlichen Fakultät der Universität Basel auf Antrag der Herren:

Prof. Dr. Marcel Tanner, Prof. Dr. Michel Burnier und Prof. Dr. Heiner C. Bucher

Basel, 5. April 2005

Prof. Dr. Hans-Jakob Wirz
Dekan

Overview

Table of contents I
Table of abbreviations V

Table of contents

Acknowledgements 7
Summary 9
Zusammenfassung 12
1. Introduction 15
    1.1 Epidemiology of chronic kidney disease (CKD) 15
    1.2 Treatment options of chronic kidney disease 17
    1.3 Prevalence of anaemia in chronic kidney disease 19
    1.4 Pathogenesis and causes of renal anaemia 20
    1.5 Clinical consequences of renal anaemia 24
    1.6 Anaemia treatment in ESRD 25
    1.6.1 Erythropoiesis-stimulating agents (ESA) 25
    1.6.2 Efficacy of ESAs 27
    1.6.3 Safety and tolerability of epoetin beta 29
    1.6.4 Clinical benefits of the treatment with ESA 29
    1.7 Factors affecting response to ESAs 31
    1.8 Target haemoglobin level 33
    1.9 Summary and rationales 33
2. Objectives 35
3. Methods and baseline characteristics 36
    3.1 Objectives and design 36
    3.2 Sampling method 37
    3.3 Sample size 38
    3.4 Treatment recommendations and concomitant medications 38
    3.5 Survey methodology and data collection 39
    3.6 Statistical analysis 42
    3.7 Representativity of the "AIMS" survey 43
    3.8 Baseline characteristics 46
    3.8.1 Participating dialysis centres and treatment population 46
    3.8.2 Patient characteristics 47
    3.9 Summary 53
4. *Anaem*I*a M*anagement in dialysis patients in *S*witzerland "AIMS": Assessment of the quality of anaemia control achieved with epoetin beta in dialysis patients in Switzerland 54
    4.1 Abstract 55
    4.2 Introduction 55
    4.3 Subjects and methods 56
    4.4 Results 58
    4.4.1 Patient characteristics 58
    4.4.2 Anaemia treatment with epoetin beta 59
    4.4.3 Iron status 66
    4.4.4 Inverse relationship between epoetin dose and haemoglobin 70
    4.5 Discussion 71

5. Adherence of anaemia management in dialysis patients in Switzerland to the European Best Practice Guidelines (EBPG) for anaemia treatment in chronic kidney disease patients 75
    5.1   Abstract 76
    5.2   Introduction 76
    5.3   Subjects and methods 78
    5.4   Results 79
    5.4.1   Patient characteristics 79
    5.4.2   Haemoglobin targets for anaemia treatment 80
    5.4.3   Iron targets for anaemia treatment 83
    5.4.4   Targets for treatment of renal anaemia with ESAs 86
    5.4.5   Failure to respond to treatment 89
    5.5   Discussion 92
6. Management of anaemia in dialyzed patients in Switzerland: a survey comparing a once a week with a 2-3 times weekly administration of epoetin beta 96
    6.1   Abstract 97
    6.2   Introduction 97
    6.3   Subjects and methods 98
    6.4   Results 100
    6.4.1   Patient characteristics 100
    6.4.2   Efficacy of the 1x weekly dosing scheme of epoetin beta 102
    6.4.3   Safety parameters 106
    6.5   Discussion 108
7. Individualizing anaemia management in dialysis patients in Switzerland – Do co-morbidities and patients' health influence physicians' target haemoglobin? 111
    7.1   Abstract 112
    7.2   Introduction 112
    7.3   Subjects and methods 114
    7.4   Results 115
    7.4.1   Patient characteristics 115
    7.4.2   Prevalence of causes and co-morbidities in dialysis patients in Switzerland 115
    7.4.3   Influence of co-morbidities on haemoglobin and physicians' target haemoglobin 119
    7.5   Discussion 123
8. Conclusions and recommendations 127
    8.1   Background and objectives 127
    8.2   Methodology 127
    8.3   Key results and lessons learnt 128
    8.4   Conclusions and outlook 130
9. Personal remarks 132
10. References 133
11. List of tables 143
12. List of figures 144
13. Appendix 146
Curriculum vitae 151

Table of abbreviations

ACE-I	angiotensin-converting enzyme inhibitor
ACORD	Anaemia Correction in Diabetes (trial)
AIMS	*A*naem*I*a *M*anagement in dialysis patients in *S*witzerland (survey)
Art.	article
AT_1-receptor antagoist	Angiotensin receptor antagonist
AUC	area under the curve
AV fistula	arterio-venous fistula
BFU-E	burst-forming unit-erythroid
CA	carcinoma
CAD	coronary artery disease
CAPD	continuous ambulatory peritoneal dialysis
CFU-E	colony-forming unit-erythroid
CH	Switzerland
CHF	congestive heart failure
CHO	Chinese hamster ovary
CHUV	Centre Hospitalier Universitaire Vaudois
CKD	chronic kidney disease
Cl	confidence interval
CO_2	carbon dioxide
COPD	chronic obstructive pulmonary disease
CREATE	*C*ardiovascular *R*isk reduction by *E*arly *A*naemia *T*reatment with *E*poetin beta (trial)
CRF	chronic renal failure
CsA	ciclosporine
CVD	cardiovascular disease
Diab	diabetes
DMMS	*D*ialysis *M*orbidity and *M*ortality *S*tudy
DN	diabetic nephropathy
DNA	desoxyribonucleid acid
EBPG	European Best Practice Guidelines for the management of anaemia in patients with chronic renal failure
EMEA	European Medicine Agency
EPO, epoetin	recombinant human erythropoetin
ERA-EDTA	European Renal Association – European Dialysis and Transplant Association
ESA	erythropoiesis-stimulating agents (epoetin alfa, epoetin beta, darbepoetin alfa)
ESAM	*E*uropean *S*urvey in *A*naemia *M*anagement
ESRD	end-stage renal disease
ex.	for example
FDA	US Food and Drug Administration
Fe	ferrum
GFR	glomerular filtration rate (ml/min); normal value: 120ml/min
GN	glomerulonephritis
h	hour
Hb	haemoglobin (g/dl)
Hct	haematocrit (%)
HCUG / HUG	Hôpital Cantonal Universitaire de Genève
HD	haemodialysis
HF	heart failure

HT	hypertension
IKS	Interkantonale Kontrollstelle für Heilmittel (now Swissmedic)
IN	interstitial nephritis
IU	international units
IU/kg/week	international units per kilogram body weight per week
i.v.	intravenous
Kt/V	measurement of the dialysis quality. Urea-dialysis dose in respect of the body mass (recommended Kt/V>1.3)
LOCF	last observation carried forward
LVEF	left ventricular ejection fraction
LVH	left ventricular hypertrophy
Misc	miscellaneous
mRNA	messenger ribonucleic acid
n	number
N/A	not applicable
NESP	novel erythropoiesis stimulation protein
NKF-K/DOQI	National Kidney Foundation and Kidney Disease Outcome Qualitiy Initiative
n.s.	not significant
NYHA	New York Heart Association
O_2	oxygen
PD	peritoneal dialysis
PEB	Praxiserfahrungsbericht (survey)
PKD	polycystic kidney disease
PN	pyelonephritis
PRCA	pure red-cell aplasia
PRESAM	*Pre*-dialysis *S*urvey on *A*naemia *M*anagement
PTH	parathormon
PVD	polyvascular disease
RBC	red blood cells
REP	rapport d'expérience pratique (survey)
rhEPO/rHuEPO	recombinant human erythropoetin
RNA	ribonucleic acid
RVD	renal vascular disease
s.c.	subcutaneous
SD	standard deviation
SGIM	Swiss Society of Internal Medicine (Schweizerische Gesellschaft für Innere Medizin)
SmPC	Summary of Product Characteristics
STI	Swiss Tropical Institute
SVK	Schweizerischer Verband für Gemeinschaftsaufgaben der Krankenversicherer
Tmax	time to maximum concentration
TNF	tumour necrosis factor
TRESAM	*Tr*ansplant *E*uropean *S*urvey on *A*naemia *M*anagement
TsF, TSAT	transferrin saturation (%)
Tx	transplantation
US	United States
USRDS	United States Renal Data System
VD	vascular disease
vs	versus
Vss	volume of distribution (ml/kg)
WHO	World Health Organization
*	significant difference

Acknowledgements

My sincerest thanks are addressed to Prof. Michel Burnier, Head of the Department of Nephrology and internal medicine, Centre Hospitalier Universitaire Vaudois (CHUV), Lausanne, who accepted to supervise my work, and to Prof. Marcel Tanner, Head of the Swiss Tropical Institute, Department of Public Health and Epidemiology in Basel, who accepted to perform the thesis at his department.

I gratefully thank Prof. Michel Burnier for all his support concerning the realization of this work. He was mainly responsible for the design, the rationale and the present structure of the thesis. I deeply appreciated the collaboration with Prof. Michel Burnier, since he was always available for stimulating discussions and gave fresh impetus for new and creative ideas. He constantly provided me with the strongest support I could have ever wished and his guidance, support and confidence enabled me to complete this work. I could also profit from his broad scientific knowledge and experience in many fields and I appreciated his sense of humour.

My thanks go also to Prof. Marcel Tanner, who gave me the possibility to perform my thesis at the Swiss Tropical Institute (STI) in Basel. I appreciated the friendly and warm reception at his department and the encouraging discussions which I experienced during my work. I could not only profit from his scientific expertise, but also from his human nature. Likewise, I thank Dr Daniela Roncari for helpful advice and information about her experience made during the doctoral degree at the STI.

Furthermore, I express my gratitude to Prof. Heiner C. Bucher, Head of the Institute of Clinical Epidemiology, Universitätsspital, Basel who accepted to be the co-referent of this thesis. I thank him for his personal interest, the open-minded discussions and for carefully looking through my work.

The idea to write a thesis came from Prof. Hans Kummer, at that time Head of the Ethical Committee at the Universitätsspital, Basel. During a discussion held about a survey in anaemic patients, he encouraged me to write a thesis based on that project.

The work would not have been possible without the support of Roche Pharma (Switzerland) Ltd, which allowed me to use the survey data in the scope of this thesis. Many thanks are addressed to my former superiors at Roche, Dr Thomas Rhyner and Katja Bürli who encouraged me to write a thesis in the medical field of anaemia. My thanks are kindly addressed to Beat Lieberherr and Dr Thomas Hefti, Roche Pharma (Switzerland) Ltd, for their confidence, understanding and support during my work.

Yet, the realization of the present thesis would not have been possible without the work and commitment of all participating dialysis centres and the support of the delegates of Roche Pharma (Switzerland) Ltd. I gratefully thank all participants for their great job and their tremendous support I experienced.

My thanks are also directed to Dr Denes Kiss, Kantonsspital Liestal, and Helga Irgl, who gave me valuable inputs regarding the development of the report forms. I thank Prof. Michel Burnier for his editorial assistance by publishing the first abstract of the survey at the congress of the Swiss Society of Internal Medicine (SGIM), Lausanne. I also thank Dr Denes Kiss, Kantonsspital Liestal, and Prof. Pierre-Yves Martin, Hôpital Cantonal Universitaire de Genève (HCUG), Geneva for their helpful comments in the publication of the previously mentioned abstract. I gratefully thank Dr Daniel Teta, CHUV, Lausanne, for his excellent presentation of the six months data at the SGIM congress in Lausanne and for his valuable support. My thanks are also directed to Dr Luca Gabutti for the enthusiastic discussion about his scientific work on artificial neural networks and for allowing to use the present survey data for the further development of his research models.

I am very grateful to Séverine Rutschi, Schweizerischer Verband für Gemeinschaftsaufgaben der Krankenversicherer (SVK), who provided me useful data regarding dialysis patients in Switzerland. Further, I would like to express my thanks to Dr Stephan Maack, Roche Pharma (Switzerland) Ltd, who supported me as to the conception of the data base and the data management. Thanks are also addressed to Dr Manfred Köhler and Michael Pfitzenmaier, Köhler GmbH, Freibourg i.Br. and to Dr Penelope Vounatsou, Swiss Tropical Institute, Basel, for their statistical support. Special thanks are also addressed to Claudia Rickli, RoNexus Services AG, Basel, for the appreciated linguistic suggestions and proofreading of the manuscript.

My special thanks go also to Christine Walliser, Swiss Tropical Institute, Basel, Christine De Gunten, CHUV, Lausanne and Philippe Urech, Roche Pharma (Switzerland) Ltd for their institutional support throughout my work. I gratefully thank all members of the Department of Nephrology at CHUV, Lausanne, and of the Swiss Tropical Institute, Basel, for their memorable support and for the agreeable and helpful working atmosphere. My warmest thanks are dedicated to Fabian Petrus for his interest in my work, his generous understanding and his kind and unforgettable support. I sincerely thank my mother, my deceased father and my sisters, Katja and Véronique, for their generous assistance, their care and their enocuragement.

Nathalie Lötscher

Summary

The prevalence of chronic kidney disease (CKD) is increasing all over the world. In the US, out of over 400,000 were end-stage renal disease (ESRD) patients in 2002, more than 90,000 were new ESRD patients. In most European countries, the incidence of ESRD increased over the last decade at an annual rate of 6-8%. End-stage renal disease is in more than 90% of the patients associated with anaemia. Untreated anaemia impairs the patients' quality of life and may be associated with the development of cardiovascular complications and reduce long-term survival. Earlier, treatment options of renal anaemia were essentially restricted to blood transfusions. The introduction of the recombinant human erythropoietin (rHuEPO, epoetin, EPO) more than ten years ago revolutionized the anaemia management. The correction of anaemia improved the prognosis of dialysis patients in terms of quality of life, cardiovascular morbidity and mortality.

Based on evidence and clinical experience, the treatment of renal anaemia slightly changed over the last decade and clinical practice varied across Europe. Therefore, the European Renal Association/European Dialysis and Transplantation Association (ERA-EDTA) developed together with European nephrologists guidelines for the treatment of renal anaemia. The European Best Practice Guidelines (EBPG) for the management of anaemia in patients with chronic renal failure was issued in 1999 with the aim to standardize anaemia management, to provide evidence-based recommendations and to improve patient care. However, more important than the publication of guidelines is their implementation in everyday clinical practice.

The present survey, *A*naem*I*a *M*anagement in dialysis patients in *S*witzerland, called "AIMS" was the first survey performed in Switzerland assessing current anaemia management in dialysis patients after the edition of the EBPG. The objectives of the survey were to assess the quality of anaemia management with epoetin beta achieved in Swiss dialysis centres and to compare it with current guidelines. Likewise, the efficacy and safety of the 1x weekly administration of epoetin beta was examined. Anaemia management in respect of the patients' clinical condition was investigated in comparison to the recommendations of the guidelines. Furthermore, it was assessed whether physicians individualize anaemia management according to the patients' clinical condition. In order to meet these objectives, no randomized clinical trial was necessary. Therefore, a practice based, open-intervention survey was performed, since no specific interference in treatment strategies was requested. Surveys of non-interventional design and with less rigid inclusion criteria may allow higher external validity of the study results. The survey was initiated in June 2002 and patient recruitment lasted until December 2003 with an observation period of 12 months. A representative patient population of 368 dialysis patients of 28 Swiss dialysis centres were included in this survey, with 340 patients from 26 centres being eligible. Of these, six-months results were presented.

The aim of this survey was to assess current anaemia management with epoetin beta in dialysis patients for 12 months. Therefore, epoetin beta therapy and efficacy parameters were requested to be documented monthly. At patient registration (baseline), aetiology of chronic renal failure, concomitant diseases, selected dialysis treatment modalities, dry weight and laboratory parameter, such as haemoglobin, serum ferritin, transferrin saturation and serum creatinine were registered. Laboratory parameters were documented if performed in the course of the clinical routine.

The main characteristics of the included patients were as follow: mean age was 64 ± 15 years and 95% of the patients were treated by haemodialysis. Most common diagnoses of end-stage renal disease were glomerulonephritis (23%), diabetic nephropathy (21%), hypertension and vascular causes (21%), and polycystic kidney disease (8%). Most prevalent baseline co-morbidities in this survey were cardiac-related. Hypertension occurred in 61% of the patients, coronary artery disease in 26% and heart failure in 17%. Diabetes was reported in 27% of the patients.

In the first analysis, the quality of anaemia control achieved with epoetin beta in dialysis patients in Switzerland was assessed. Six months results demonstrated a high standard of anaemia management in the participating dialysis centres. Mean haemoglobin concentration was 11.8 ± 1.4 g/dl at baseline and 11.8 ± 1.4 g/dl at month 6 and remained stable over the total observation period. 74% and at 76% of the patients achieved haemoglobin concentration of ≥11 g/dl at baseline and month 6 (overall 79%), respectively. Mean weekly epoetin dose administered was 143 ± 108 IU/kg/week at baseline and 155 ± 126 IU/kg/week at month 6. The findings of "AIMS" suggest that anaemia management improved over the last five years towards higher haemoglobin concentrations in dialysis patients compared to the results in the "ESAM" survey.

In the second analysis, anaemia management of dialysis patients in Swiss dialysis centres was compared to the recommendations of the EBPG. Further, physicians' targets for anaemia treatment were assessed in respect of the guidelines and of the achieved values. Anaemia management in dialysis patients in Switzerland corresponded for the majority of the patients to the European guidelines and was well controlled. Physicians' target for haemoglobin concentrations tended towards 12 g/dl, 60% of the participating centres aimed at partial normalization (Hb ≥12 g/dl) and 23% at full normalization (Hb ≥13 g/dl) of haemoglobin conentration in dialysis patients. The physicians' target haemoglobin level was achieved in only 48% of the patients compared to 79% achieving 11 g/dl, since physicians' goals were ambitious with a trend towards normalized haemoglobin concentrations. In contrast to the recommendation, 90% of the patients received epoetin beta already at therapy initiation as a 1x weekly dosing regimen and 65% of all patients with intravenous epoetin administration received epoetin beta as a 1x weekly dosing scheme, even though there is lack of evidence to support 1x weekly dosing of intravenous epoetin in haemodialysis patients. These findings demonstrate that clinical practice diverges partially from the recommended guidelines.

In the third analysis the efficacy and safety of two dosing schedules of epoetin beta in dialysis patients were compared. The 1x weekly subcutaneous administration of epoetin beta in stable chronic kidney disease patients was approved in 2001 by the European Authority and, therefore, one of the objectives of the survey was to elaborate the relevance of the 1x weekly administration in Swiss dialysis centres. 61% (n=207) of the patients received epoetin beta 1x weekly for all six months and 39% (n=133) received it 2-3x weekly. Baseline parameters of both groups were comparable with the exception of age and baseline dose of epoetin beta. The 1x weekly administration of epoetin beta appeared to be as effective as the 2-3x weekly administration in maintaining haemoglobin concentration. These data show that in a large proportion of dialysis patients anaemia can be effectively managed with a 1x weekly administration of epoetin beta, reducing thus the work-load for medical staff.

In the fourth analysis, the prevalence of diagnosis and co-morbidities and the impact of co-morbidities on anaemia treatment were assessed in dialysis patients in Switzerland. The prevalence of the most common diagnosis and co-morbidities of Swiss dialysis patients corresponded to those of the ERA-EDTA registry and of the USRDS registry, respectively. The influence of the underlying disease on haemoglobin and epoetin dose was investigated. In the univariate and multivariate analysis, diabetes and heart failure showed to have a significant influence on patients' haemoglobin concentration. Mean haemoglobin was highest in patients with COPD (chronic obstructive pulmonary disease) and lowest in cancer patients. The majority of the dialysis centres aimed at identical target haemoglobin concentrations for all dialysis patients, irrespective of the co-morbidities or the physical condition. Only 40% of all dialysis centres said to individualize anaemia treatment.

The present survey provided evidence about the quality of anaemia management in Swiss dialysis patients for the first time after the publication of the EBPG in 1998. The findings of "AIMS" demonstrate that a high quality of anaemia control in dialysis patients in Switzerland was achieved. Target haemoglobin concentrations in Switzerland tended towards 12 g/dl and higher, reflecting the ongoing discussion about the optimal target haemoglobin level in dialysis patients which has not been defined yet. Anaemia treatment in Swiss dialysis centres was in adherence to current guidelines and was tailored to the patients' health in approximately one third of all participating dialysis centres. In order to improve patient care, registry database and quality assessment tools have been increasingly used in many clinical disciplines. Up to now, no registry database has been established for renal patients in Switzerland. The increasing age of dialysis patients and the number of associated co-morbidities make the management of these patients more complex. Quality assessement tools are becoming more and more essential in order to improve patient care and therapy on an individual base. The present survey represents a simplified tool to perform quality assessments of anaemia management in chronic kidney disease patients in each dialysis centre and may build the basis for the national registry database.

Zusammenfassung

Die Zahl der Patienten mit chronischer Niereninsuffizienz steigt weltweit an. Inzwischen leiden über 400'000 Personen in den USA an einer Niereninsuffizienz, wobei jährlich mehr als 90'000 neue Patienten diagnostiziert werden. Eine ähnliche Entwicklung ist auch in Europa zu beobachten, wobei die jährliche Inzidenzrate zwischen 6-8% beträgt. Eine terminale Niereninsuffizienz ist in mehr als 90% der Fälle von einer Anämie begleitet, die unbehandelt die Lebensqualität dieser Patienten beträchtlich beeinflusst und zu kardiovaskulären Komplikationen sowie zu einem verminderten Langzeitüberleben führt. Die Einführung von Erythropoetin (rHuEPO, Epoetin, EPO) vor mehr als zehn Jahren war ein wichtiger Meilenstein in der Behandlung der renalen Anämie. Durch die Behandlung der renalen Anämie mit Epoetin konnte sowohl die Lebensqualität als auch die Prognose der Dialysepatienten wesentlich verbessert werden.

Die Behandlung der renalen Anämie hat sich während der letzten zehn Jahre aufgrund klinischer Erfahrungen und neuer Erkenntnisse laufend verändert. Teilweise konnten beträchtliche Unterschiede bei der Anämiebehandlung zwischen den einzelnen Ländern festgestellt werden. Deshalb hat die European Renal Association/European Dialysis and Transplantation Association (ERA-EDTA) gemeinsam mit Nephrologen aus verschiedenen europäischen Ländern evidenzgestützte Richtlinien zur Behandlung der renalen Anämie entwickelt. Die europäischen Richtlinien zur Behandlung der Anämie bei chronischer Niereninsuffizienz (European Best Practice Guidelines [EBPG]) wurden erstmals 1999 herausgegeben mit dem Ziel, die Anämietherapie bei Niereninsuffizienz zu standardisieren und die Behandlung der Patienten zu verbessern.

Der vorliegende Praxiserfahrungsbericht - *AnaemIa Management in dialysis patients in Switzerland* „AIMS" - war der erste Praxiserfahrungsbericht, der die aktuelle Anämiebehandlung bei Dialysepatienten grossflächig nach dem Erscheinen der EBPG in der Schweiz untersuchte. Die Untersuchung hatte zum Ziel, die Qualität der Anämietherapie mit Epoetin beta in Schweizer Dialysezentren zu untersuchen und mit den aktuellen Richtlinien der Anämiebehandlung (EBPG) zu vergleichen. In der folgenden Analyse wurde der Stellenwert sowie die Wirksamkeit und Sicherheit der 1x wöchentlichen Verabreichung von Epoetin beta untersucht. Im Weiteren wurde untersucht, ob die Anämietherapie bei Dialysepatienten individuell gestaltet und aufgrund von zugrundeliegenden Grund- bzw. Begleiterkrankung adaptiert wird. Die vorgenannten Fragestellungen können in Form eines Praxiserfahrungsberichtes untersucht werden, ohne dass eine aufwändige randomisierte klinische Studie notwendig wird. Da aufgrund der Untersuchungsziele keine Intervention in der Behandlung der Anämie notwendig war, wurden die Erhebungen mittels eines Praxiserfahrungsberichtes gewonnen. Erhebungen im Rahmen von Praxiserfahrungsberichten weisen im Vergleich zu Studien meist eine höhere externe Validität auf; dies aufgrund ihres nicht-interventionellen Charakters. Nachteilig für diese Art der Erhebung sind Verzerrungen (bias), die auftreten können. Die Patienten, die im Rahmen von „AIMS" eingeschlossen wurden, waren für die Dialysepopulation der Schweiz repräsentativ. Der Praxiserfahrungsbericht wurde im Juni 2002 gestartet, mit der Möglichkeit, Dialysepatienten bis Ende Dezember 2003 einzuschliessen. Die Beobachtungsdauer betrug 12 Monate. Insgesamt wurden 368 Dialysepatienten von 28 Dialysestationen (repräsentative Patientenpopulation) in den Praxiserfahrungsbericht eingeschlossen, wovon 340 Patienten aus 26 Dialysezentren auswertbar waren. In dieser Arbeit wurden die Sechs-Monats-Daten ausgewertet und diskutiert.

Ziel des Praxiserfahrungsberichtes war es, die aktuelle Anämiebehandlung von Dialysepatienten mit Epoetin beta über einen Zeitraum von 12 Monaten zu untersuchen. Dabei wurden die Behandlung mit Epoetin beta sowie die wichtigsten Parameter monatlich dokumentiert. Bei der Patientenanmeldung wurden nebst der Dialysemethode, der Diagnose und den Begleiterkrankungen der chronischen Niereninsuffizienz folgende weitere Parameter erhoben: Trockengewicht, Hämoglobin, Serumferritin, Transferrinsättigung und Serumkreatinin. Die Laborparameter waren insofern zu dokumentieren, als sie im Rahmen des klinischen Alltags erhoben wurden.

Das mittlere Alter der Patienten betrug 64 ± 15 Jahre, wovon 95% mittels Hämodialyse behandelt wurden. Die häufigsten Diagnosen der chronischen Niereninsuffizienz waren Glomerulonephritis (23%), diabetische Nephropathie (21%), Hypertonie sowie vaskuläre Ursachen (21%) und Zystennieren (8%). Die häufigsten Begleiterkrankungen waren kardiovaskulär bedingt. Eine Hypertonie trat bei 61%, koronare Herzkrankheit bei 26% und eine Herzinsuffizienz bei 17% der eingeschlossenen Patienten auf.

In der ersten Analyse wurde die Qualität der Anämietherapie unter Epoetin beta bei Dialysepatienten in der Schweiz untersucht. Die Ergebnisse der Sechs-Monats-Daten zeigen, dass die partizipierenden Dialysezentren einen hohen Qualitätsstandard in der Anämiebehandlung erzielt haben. Der Hämoglobinwert blieb während der gesamten Beobachtungsdauer äusserst stabil und war bei Patientenanmeldung 11,8 ± 1,4 g/dl und betrug nach sechs Monaten 11,8 ± 1,4 g/dl. Bei Patientenanmeldung und nach Monat 6 erreichten 74% bzw. 76% der Patienten einen Hämoglobinwert ≥11 g/dl bei einer mittleren Epoetin-Wochendosis von 143 ± 108 IE/kg/Woche bzw. 155 ± 126 IE/kg/Woche. Im Weiteren konnte gezeigt werden, dass sich die Anämiebehandlung und somit die Hämoglobinwerte im Verlaufe der letzten fünf Jahre wesentlich verbesserten verglichen mit den Resultaten der „ESAM" Studie.

In der zweiten Analyse wurde die Anämiebehandlung der Dialysepatienten in der Schweiz mit den aktuellen Empfehlungen der EBPG verglichen. Die Ziel-Hämoglobinwerte der jeweiligen Zentren sollten mit den aktuellen Empfehlungen und den erreichten Hämoglobinwerten verglichen werden. Die Untersuchung ergab, dass die Anämiebehandlung bei Dialysepatienten in der Schweiz sich nach den internationalen Empfehlungen richtet und gut kontrolliert war. Die Ziel-Hämoglobinwerte lagen bei einer Mehrheit der Ärzte bei 12 g/dl. 60% der teilnehmenden Dialysezentren gaben an, den Hämoglobin-Wert ihrer Dialysepatienten teilweise (Hb=12 g/dl) und 23% vollständig (Hb=13 g/dl) zu normalisieren. 48% der Patienten erreichten die Ziel-Hämoglobinwerte der Nephrologen, wobei 79% den Ziel-Hämoglobinwert von 11 g/dl erreichten. Dies, weil teilweise sehr hohe Zielwerte angestrebt wurden, die praktisch einer vollständigen Anämiekorrektur gleichkamen. Im Gegensatz zu den Empfehlungen erhielten bereits 90% der Epoetin-naïven Patienten zur Therapiestart Epoetin beta als 1x wöchentliche Gabe. Bei 65% der Patienten mit intravenöser Verabreichung wurde Epoetin beta ebenfalls 1x wöchentlich verabreicht, obwohl hierfür wissenschaftliche Grundlagen fehlten. Die Ergebnisse zeigen auch, dass Empfehlungen nicht immer im klinischen Alltag umgesetzt und angewendet werden.

In der dritten Analyse wurde die Wirksamkeit und die Sicherheit zweier Dosierungsschemen von Epoetin beta bei Dialysepatienten miteinander verglichen. Die 1x wöchentliche subkutane Verabreichung von Epoetin beta an stabil eingestellte Patienten mit renaler Anämie wurde 2001 von der Europäischen Behörde (EMEA) registriert. Eine der Zielsetzungen war, den Stellenwert der 1x wöchentlichen Verabreichung von Epoetin beta in Schweizer Dialysezentren nach Indikationserweiterung zu untersuchen. Die Resultate zeigen, dass 61% (n=207) der Patienten über 6 Monate mit der 1x wöchentlichen Gabe von Epoetin beta behandelt wurden und 39% (n=133) mit der 2-3x wöchentlichen Gabe. Die Grundparameter beider Gruppen waren bei Patienteneinschluss (Baseline) vergleichbar, mit Ausnahme des Alters und der Anfangsdosierung von Epoetin beta. Die 1x wöchentliche Dosierung von Epoetin beta schien gleich wirksam zu sein, wie die auf 2-3 Wochengaben aufgeteilte Wochendosis von Epoetin beta. Die Anämie kann somit bei einer Mehrzahl der Dialysepatienten effektiv mit einer 1x wöchentlichen Verabreichung von Epoetin beta behandelt werden, was zusätzlich den Arbeitsaufwand für das Medizinalpersonal reduziert.

Die vierte Analyse befasste sich mit der Prävalenz von Diagnosen und Begleiterkrankungen von Dialysepatienten in der Schweiz. Ferner wurde der mögliche Einfluss von Begleiterkrankungen auf die Anämiebehandlung bei Dialysepatienten untersucht. Die Diagnosen sowie die Begleiterkrankungen der Dialysepatienten aus der Schweiz waren in ihrer Häufigkeit mit denjenigen der ERA-EDTA-Datenbank bzw. der USRDS-Datenbank vergleichbar. In einer univariaten sowie multivariaten Analyse wurde der Einfluss von zugrundeliegenden Erkrankungen auf die Hämoglobinkonzentration und die Epoetindosis untersucht. Dabei zeigte sich, dass Diabetes und Herzinsuffizienz einen signifikanten Einfluss auf den Hämoglobinwert hatten. Die höchsten Hämoglobinwerte wurden bei Patienten mit COPD und die tiefsten bei Patienten mit Tumorerkrankungen gemessen. Die Mehrzahl der Dialysestationen strebten für alle Dialysepatienten die gleichen Zielhämoglobinwerte an, unabhängig von Begleit- oder Grunderkrankungen. Nur etwa 40% der Dialysestationen gaben an, die Anämiebehandlung bei Dialysepatienten individuell und je nach Gesundheitszustand des Patienten anzupassen.

Die Untersuchung liefert erstmals nach der Publikation der EBPG von 1998 wertvolle Erkenntnisse zur aktuellen Anämiebehandlung bei Dialysepatienten in der Schweiz. Die Ergebnisse zeigen, dass ein hoher Standard in der Anämiebehandlung bei Dialysepatienten in der Schweiz erzielt wurde. Die Mehrzahl der Ärzte (Nephrologen) strebten Ziel-Hämoglobinwerte von gegen 12 g/dl und höher bei Dialysepatienten an. Ausserdem konnte aufgezeigt werden, dass sich die aktuelle Anämiebehandlung in der Schweiz mehrheitlich nach den Empfehlungen der EPBG richtet und sie bei einem Drittel der Dialysestationen individuell auf den Patienten massgeschneidert angepasst erfolgt. Bis heute gibt es in der Schweiz noch keine Datenbank für Patienten mit Niereninsuffizienz wie in anderen Ländern. Aufgrund des zunehmenden Alters und der Vielzahl von Begleiterkrankungen bei Dialysepatienten wird deren Behandlung immer komplexer. Um diesem Anspruch gerecht zu werden, wird eine regelmässige Qualitätsdokumentation und –beurteilung immer notwendiger, um die Patientenbetreuung zu verbessern und auch individuellen Behandlungsmöglichkeiten zum Wohle des Patienten eine bessere Entscheidungsgrundlage zu geben. Der vorliegende Praxiserfahrungsbericht stellt ein einfaches Instrument zur Beurteilung der Qualität der Anämiebehandlung bei chronischen Nierenpatienten dar, das in jedem Dialysezentrum einsetzbar ist und als Basis zum Aufbau einer nationalen Datenbank dienen kann.

1. Introduction

Chronic renal disease continues to increase in prevalence and incidence. Registry data reveal some 300,000 patients on dialysis in both Europe and the United States; 60,000 new patients start dialysis each year in Europe and 80,000 in the United States [1]. The two most common causes of end-stage renal failure are diabetes (mostly type 2) and hypertension, followed by glomerulonephritis and interstitial nephritis [2].

Chronic renal disease is a multifactor progressive disease where increasing nephron damage impairs the glomerular filtration rate (GFR) and causes uraemia. End-stage renal disease patient (Stage IV: GFR < 10 ml/min) requires renal replacement therapy, either dialysis or transplantation. A frequent complication, present in over 90% of dialysis patients, is renal anaemia. It begins in the early stages of the disease and worsens in correlation with the decline in renal function. The prevalence of anaemia in chronic kidney disease is inversely correlated to the residual renal function. Anaemia has been identified as an independent risk factor for left ventricular hypertrophy, since it increases cardiac morbidity and mortality [3]. The main cause of renal anaemia is erythropoietin (EPO) deficiency. The kidneys fail to synthesize adequate quantities of EPO to support haematopoiesis [4-7]. The treatment of anaemia was revolutionized over 15 years ago by the introduction of epoetin, which is now administered to 90% of dialysis patients and 30% of patients in pre-dialysis renal failure [8].

Anaemia treatment with epoetin for chronic kidney disease (CKD) patients results in numerous benefits:

Non-cardiovascular benefits [9, 10]
- improved quality of life: decreased fatigue and depression
- improved working capacity
- improved exercise tolerance.

Cardiovascular benefits [11-14]
- decreased cardiac output
- decreased left ventricular hypertrophy
- decreased overall and cardiovascular morbidity and mortality.

1.1 Epidemiology of chronic kidney disease (CKD)

The National Kidney Foundation defined in the NKF-K/DOQI guidelines (National Kidney Foundation and Kidney Disease Outcome Quality Initiative) "chronic kidney disease (CKD)" according to the following criteria: [15]
- Kidney damage existing for ≥3 months defined by structural or functional abnormalities of the kidney, with or without decreased glomerular filtration rate, (GFR) detectable by either pathological abnormalities or marker of kidney damage, including abnormalities in the composition of the blood or urine, or abnormalities in imaging test, and
- a glomerular filtration rate <60ml/min/1.73 m^2 for ≥ 3 months, with or without kidney damage.

The term "end-stage renal disease" (ESRD) is very often used because of its administrative use in the US referring to all patients treated with replacement therapy (dialysis or transplantation) irrespective of the level of kidney function. Clinically chronic kidney disease (CKD) can be classified in five stages defined by the degree of the glomerular filtration rate. Chronic kidney disease normally worsens over time and consequently the risk of adverse events or outcomes increases over time with disease severity. Glomerular filtration rate (GFR) is one of the best measuring parameters represent the degree of kidney damage.

Stage	Phase	Description	Glomerular filtration rate $(ml/min/1.73m^2)$
I	Kidney damage	Kidney damage with normal or increased GFR	≥90
II	Impaired renal function	Kidney damage with mild decrease of GFR	60-89
III	Chronic renal insufficiency	Moderate decrease of GFR	30-59
IV	Chronic renal failure	Severe decrease of GFR	15-29
V	End-stage renal failure	Kidney failure	<15

Table 1-1: Stages of chronic kidney disease classified by glomerular filtration rate

There is a great inter-individual variety in the severity of the symptoms of uraemia and the progression of chronic kidney disease. At the beginning of chronic kidney disease, patients are generally free from symptoms but most of them are hypertensive. A decline of GFR below 45 ml/min increases the symptoms of tiredness in these patients, influences their well-being and decreases the working capacity. Anaemia and metabolic abnormalities (metabolic acidosis and disturbances of calcium and phosphorus metabolism) may be present when GFR falls below 30 ml/min. Additional symptoms such as nausea, vomiting, gastritis and cardiovascular symptoms, congestive heart failure, neurological symptoms and oedema may occur in patients with further decline of the GFR (GFR <15 ml/min). Regardless of the underlying disease, chronic kidney disease is characterized by a continuous loss of renal function with a linear decline in glomerular filtration rate and a hyperbolic increase in serum creatinine.

Diabetes is the leading cause of end-stage renal disease. Diabetes is in about 45% among all incident and in 35% of all prevalent end-stage renal disease patients in the US the responsible cause. The prevalence of diabetes as primary diagnosis of ESRD in the US was almost twice as high as in European countries, i.e. Belgium, Denmark and Sweden. A possible explanation might be the higher proportion of obese patients in USA than in Europe. Obesity is a major risk factor for the development of diabetes type II. Recent studies indicate that the incidence rate of diabetes is still rising, with recent estimates of 7-9% in Europe and the US [1] [16-18]. Hypertension (27%) and glomerular diseases (11%) are the second and third common causes of kidney failure in incident new end-stage renal disease patients in the US [1]. Approximately 10% of all dialysis patients have polycystic kidney disease, which is the most common hereditary kidney disease.

The distribution of the causes of ESRD by demographic subgroup showed that causes of ESRD vary depending on age. In young ESRD patients (< 20 years old) the most frequent diagnoses are glomerulonephritis (30%) and cystic/hereditary/congenital diseases (26%). Diabetes is very rare in young patients in contrast to older patients where diabetes and hypertension are the most common causes of ESRD.

Diabetic kidney disease usually follows a characteristic clinical course after the onset of diabetes, beginning with a silent phase with basically normal renal function for the first 10-15 years followed by the clinically manifest phase characterized as a steady decline in glomerular filtration rate and a steady increase in microalbuminuria leading to end-stage renal failure after 15-30 years [19].

Stage	Albuminuria	Blood pressure	GFR (ml/min)*	Years
Hyperfunction	absent	normal	increased	Onset of diabetes
Latent	absent	normal	high normal	
Incipient nephropathy	30-300 mg/24h	rising	failing	5-15
Clinically manifest nephropathy	>300 mg/24h	elevated	failing	10-15
Renal failure	high	elevated	reduced	15-30

*GFR = Glomerular filtration rate, normal = 120ml/min

Table 1-2: Stages of diabetic nephropathy after Morgenson [19]

1.2 Treatment options of chronic kidney disease

End-stage renal patients require renal replacement therapy. Two treatment modalities of renal replacement are available beside renal transplantation, namely haemodialysis and peritoneal dialysis. Dialysis treatment removes nitrogenous and other waste products, corrects the electrolytes balance, water and acid base abnormalities associated with renal failure, however, dialysis does not correct the endocrine abnormalities associated with the kidney dysfunction. The purpose of dialysis is to achieve a long patient survival and a good quality of life and to reduce secondary end-organ damage due to uraemia [20].

Haemodialysis (HD)

The basic principle of haemodialysis is the diffusion of solutes across a semi-permeable. Blood and dialysate solutions are transported in opposite directions across a separated semi-permeable membrane, which allows an exchange of corporal toxins (uric acid, urea) and corporal fluid. The greater the concentration gradient across the semi-permeable membrane the higher the diffusion rate and the better the removal of urea and creatinine and the replenishment of serum bicarbonate [20, 21].

In haemodialysis patients, toxins and excess of corporal fluid are removed by means of a dialyser (artificial extra-corporal kidney) from the patient's body. For this purpose a vascular access is needed which allows to remove 300-400 ml blood per minute. The development of the "Scribner-Shunt" made haemodialysis first practicable for chronic use. An important progress was achieved in 1966 with the introduction of the arterio-venous fistula (AV-fistula) which is used in most dialysis patient [21]. Haemodialysis is generally performed three times a week for 3 or 4 hours in hospitals or in dialysis centres. In Switzerland, approximately 2,800 patients are treated with haemodialysis, which is generally performed in hospitals in a three times weekly rhythm [22].

In recently published studies dialysis was performed in a daily rhythm either during night or as a short daytime, which appeared to be superior to any other currently available treatment for heamodialysis patients in terms of clearance, dialysis quality, clinical conditions and patients' outcome [23-25]. Short-time daily haemodialysis may be more convenient for patients at work, young and mobile patients, in that it minimize the interference in the patients' social and work life. Three times weekly haemodialysis may be more adequate for elderly, disable patients, reducing time-consuming conveyance and allowing one-day recovery between the dialysis.

Peritoneal dialysis (PD)

Peritoneal dialysis was developed in the 1970s based on assuming that the high concentration of glucose fluid installed in the abdominal cavity can maintain urea in equilibrium. While in haemodialysis the exchange between blood und dialysate solutions is performed through a semi-permeable membrane as an extracorporal circulation, in peritoneal dialysis the peritoneum is used as an alternative membrane surface. For PD a permanent catheter is inserted into the abdominal cavity. Dialysis fluid is instilled into the cavity and remains several hours in the peritoneum. Fluid is removed through osmotic ultrafiltration by use of hypertonic dialysate solutions. Small substances, such as urea, equilibrate rapidly between plasma and dialysate. During the long dwell time of PD, larger molecules, such as creatinine, are dialysed continuously, due to the concentration gradient throughout the dwell time [21, 26].

The most common PD method is the continuous ambulatory peritoneal dialysis (CAPD) where dialysate (mostly hypertonic glucose fluid) is rapidly infused into the cavity with a dwell time of 4-6 hours, then the exceeding accumulated volume is removed and the dialysate is exchanged by the patient. A standard CAPD regimen consists of 2 litres exchanges, four times daily, three during the day and one over night. The most common complication of the peritoneal dialysis method is peritonitis due to bacterial contaminations [3, 21, 26]. CAPD gained broad acceptance as an alternative method of renal replacement therapy for patients with end-stage renal disease, providing a larger autonomy to patients with lower costs compared to haemodialysis. CAPD is often used in patients who prefer the independence of self-care and in those who have difficulty with vascular access. However, peritoneal dialysis is used in approximately 10% of all dialysis patients, with a worldwide stagnation or even a decline [27-30].

Transplantation

In Switzerland, the number of solid organ transplantation decreased form 424 to 410 in 2002 and increased in 2003 up to 491 again. Kidney transplantation was performed in 299 patients in Switzerland in 2003 compared to 225 in 2002 [22]. A stagnation of kidney transplantation was observed over the last decade despite intensive educational campaigns all over Europe [28]. For this reason, an increase of the proportion of transplantated patients is not expected.

The first successful transplantation was performed in 1954 by Merrill and Murray as a living donation between identical twins. Renal transplantation for nonidentical twins also became reality during the 1960s, because of the introduction of the first immunosuppressive therapy. The kidney transplantation is nowadays a well established alternative opportunity for renal replacement. A successful transplantation is the only renal replacement modality which leads to a full normalization of the kidney function. Kidney transplantation offers a higher degree of autonomy to the patients compared to dialysis. As a disadvantage, transplanted patients require the intake of immunosuppressive medicine for the rest of their life, which can provoke undesirable adverse events but are necessary to prevent the rejection of the transplanted organ.

The survival rate in transplanted patients is generally higher than in dialysis patients. The one year survival was 83% in dialysis patients (incident dialysis patients, unadjusted) compared to 94% in transplanted patients (cadaver donors, unadjusted). The discrepancies between transplanted and dialyzed patients were even greater for two and five years survival rates. The two year and five year survival rate was 69.4% and 37.6% in dialysis and 91.9% and 83.8% in transplanted patients in Europe, respectively [28].

In conclusion, haemodialysis is the most common dialysis treatment in the US and in European countries. In 2001, 86,000 patients initiated haemodialysis and approximately 7,000 peritoneal dialysis, while 2,400 patients were transplanted according to the USRDS annual report of 2003. Peritoneal dialysis was observed to stagnate or to decline worldwide [30]. In Switzerland, the preferred dialysis modality is haemodialysis and reveals a similar picture to other industrialized countries. Approximately 11-12% of the dialysis patients are on peritoneal dialysis in Switzerland [22], despite the fact that peritoneal dialysis generates lower costs than haemodialysis. Peritoneal dialysis offers a higher autonomy to patients but the disadvantages are higher infection rate, peritonitis and increased burden of self-care. Kidney transplantation was performed in nearly 300 patients in 2003 in Switzerland and is a limited method of renal replacement due to the restricted availability of donors.

1.3   Prevalence of anaemia in chronic kidney disease

Anaemia in predialysis and dialysis patients

The prevalence of anaemia increases as creatinine clearance decreases [3, 31]. Anaemia normally becomes clinically manifest, when the glomerular filtration rate falls below 25 ml/min and creatinine clearance below 45 ml/min. A decrease in haemoglobin level below the normal levels (14-18 g/dl for men and 12-16 g/dl for women) starts already at an earlier stage of chronic kidney disease. Thus, in predialysis stage of chronic kidney disease, haemoglobin values can already start to decline to anaemic level in stage II or stage III [31-33]. Anaemia is defined by the World Health Organization (WHO) as a haemoglobin concentration below 13.0 g/dl for adult males and post-menopausal women, and below 12.0 g/dl for pre-menopausal women [34]. A Canadian multicentre study, using these definitions, showed that 87% of patients with chronic kidney disease did not require dialysis at a creatinine clearance of less than 25 ml/min and 25% at a creatinine clearance of more than 50 ml/min had anaemia (defined as Hb levels < 13 g/dl). At the onset of dialysis, 90% of the patients were found to have anaemia independently of the primary disease of chronic kidney disease (CKD).

Anaemia in renal transplant patients

Anaemia also occurs in renal transplant patients and is similar to that observed in chronic kidney disease patients with equal treatment recommendations. At the time of transplanttation, nearly all patients are anaemic, since dialysis patients are normally at a haemoglobin level between 11-12 g/dl. After renal transplantation, erythropoiesis begins to rise two days after transplantation, and after one year 10 to 40% of the patients remain anaemic despite having normal graft function [35, 36]. As a matter of fact, most patients achieve a normal haemoglobin concentration one year after transplantation and are not anaemic. This improvement of erythropoiesis is due to the erythropoietin production in the allograft and the loss of uraemia [37]. The prevalence of anaemia increases with time after transplantation. After five years' post-transplantation, 26% of the patients were anaemic [38]. This figure is comparable to the findings of the recent Transplant European Survey on Anaemia (TRESAM), where 38.6% of the patients were found anaemic (11.6% with moderate and 8.5% with severe anaemia) [36]. Risk factors found for post-transplant anaemia found, were CO_2 (metabolic acidosis was considered as surrogate marker for renal impairment), blood urea, nitrogen and creatinine (<2mg/dl). A strong association was also found between haemoglobin concentration and renal graft function in renal transplant patients [38].

Even though it would have been of value to assess the prevalence of anaemia in transplanted patients as well, the present survey *AnaemIa Management in dialysis patients in Switzerland* "AIMS" was restricted to dialysis patients, since the objective was to assess anaemia management in dialysis patients in Switzerland.

1.4   Pathogenesis and causes of renal anaemia

Erythropoietin deficiency appears to be the major cause of anaemia in chronic kidney disease. Serum erythropoietin level in CKD patients does not increase exponentially when haemoglobin concentration declines as compared to healthy persons. Anaemia of CKD is characterized by a relative deficiency of erythropoietin, because the serum erythropoietin level is inappropriately low for the degree of anaemia. This type of anaemia is characterised by normochromic and normocytc blood cells, and hypoplasia of erythroid cells [5, 39]. However, other factors like the following ones are also likely to be involved [15, 40]:

- Impaired erythropoiesis:
    - relative erythropoietin deficiency
    - deficiency of iron, vitamin B_{12} or folate deficiency
    - severe hyperparathyroidism or hypoparathyroidism
    - inadequacy of dialysis
    - infection
    - transfusion-induced erythroid suppression
- Shortened red cell survival
- Chronic blood loss
    - during haemodialysis
    - for diagnostics
    - gastrointestinal bleeding

Erythropoiesis

Erythropoiesis is a fundamental process of haematopoiesis which stimulates the red cell lineage in the bone marrow to produce significant haemoglobin concentration for tissue oxygenation. Erythropoiesis occurs normally in the blood-forming tissue of the bone marrow. Under conditions of anaemia or hypoxia, the red cell lineage is stimulated in order to have sufficient circulating haemoglobin to maintain adequate oxygen delivery throughout the body.

Erythropoietin is synthesized primarily in the kidney (peritubular interstitial cells of the kidney), and to a lesser degree (about 10%) in the liver. The exact formation site of the erythropoietin is not known yet [41]. The erythropoietin hormone is a glycoprotein with a molecular weight of approximately 30,400 Dalton and is composed of 165 amino acids and 4 carbohydrate chains. Normal serum erythropoietin levels range from 10-30 mU/ml and can increase 100-1,000-fold under hypoxic or anaemic conditions. The erythropoietin hormone follows the characteristic endocrine pattern of formation in one site – the kidney, transport through the blood stream, to a distant site to action – the bone marrow.

Role of erythropoietin in the erythropoiesis

The maintenance of an adequate supply of oxygen to the body tissues is vital for survival. Since to a large degree the oxygen-carrying capacity of blood is governed by the concentration of erythrocytes in the blood, appropriate regulation of erythropoiesis is crucial. The physiological pathway of erythropoietin synthesis involves a complex feedback model that is regulated by cellular oxygen concentration with the purpose to regulate red cell production (see Figure 1-1). It controls the number of circulating erythrocytes in the blood in order to maintain and to secure adequate tissue oxygenation [39, 42].

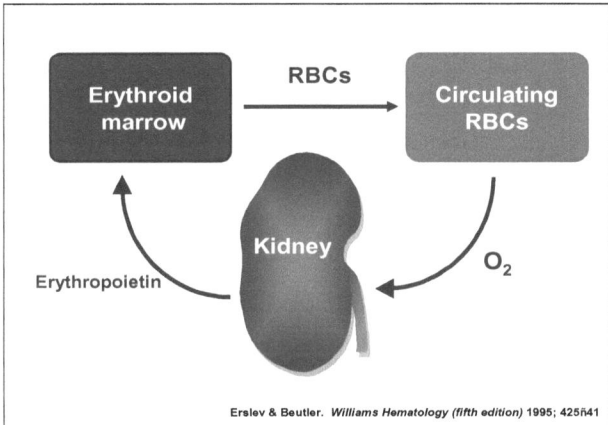

Erslev & Beutler. *Williams Hematology (fifth edition)* 1995; 425ñ41

RBC= red blood cell; O_2 = oxygen

Figure 1-1: Regulation of erythropoiesis: Feedback regulation

A decrease in the oxygen concentration induces the production of erythropoietin in the kidney. From its production site, erythropoietin gets to the bone marrow and binds to specific receptors on the erythroid cells [39, 42] and stimulates the maturation of red blood cells. Binding of erythropoietin to the receptor induces the following cascade in the maturation process of red blood cells:
- The hormone first binds to BFU-E (burst-forming unit-erythroid) cells, which are highly proliferative and require a large amount of erythropoietin to progress to the next development step (Figure 1-2).
- BFU-E cells gradually cease to multiply and enter into a critical erythropoietin-dependent colony-forming unit-erythroid (CFU-E) stage.
- CFU-E cells proliferate into erythroid precursors, are transformed to reticulocytes and become finally matured erythrocytes.

In the absence of adequate levels of erythropoietin, the CFU-E cells undergo apoptosis [43, 44]. One of the main functions of erythropoietin is the inhibition of CFU-E apoptosis, allowing these cells to mature into erythroblasts. After the red blood cells have passed from the bone marrow into the circulation, erythropoietin is responsible for their survival [15, 16].

Regulation of erythropoietin production

Erythropoietin is an essential growth and survival factor for erythroid precursor cells as previously mentioned. The number of newly formatted erythrocytes correlates directly to the plasma-erythropoietin concentration. The regulation of erythropoietin production occurs by the tissue oxygen tension (difference between oxygen supply and oxygen consumption) in the kidney and the liver. A decrease in oxygen saturation or oxygen supply capacity stimulates erythropoietin secretion (see Figure 1-2).

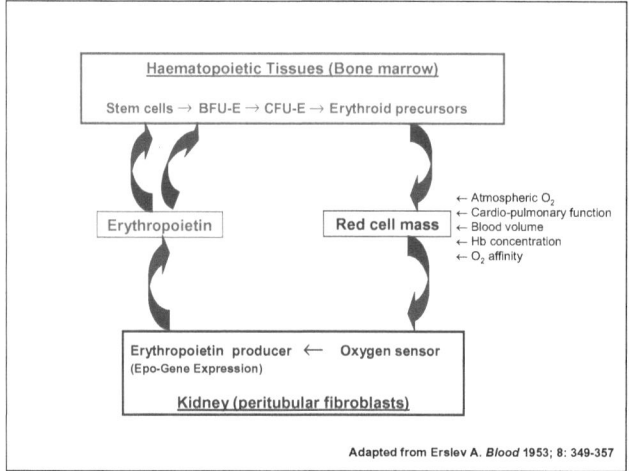

BFU-E=burst-forming unit-erythroid; CFU-E=colony-forming unit-erythroid; Hb=haemoglobin

Figure 1-2: Regulation of erythropoiesis as an oxygen-dependent feedback mechanism

The role of oxygen in the kidney is primarily to provide energy for the sodium reabsorption, which depends on the glomerular filtration rate and renal blood flow. A decrease in oxygen supply due to decreased renal blood flow, or decreased oxygen transport capacity (anaemia) accelerates erythropoietin gene expression and the production of renal mRNA.

The mechanism of how changes in oxygen supply are registered in the kidney is still not fully understood [47]. The regulation of the renal erythropoietin production is very sensitive. Healthy persons are able to compensate for increased erythropoietin requirements in order to maintain a balance between erythropoietin production and haemoglobin levels. An increase of serum erythropoietin concentration can be detected after blood transfusion. Populations living at high altitude produce a higher amount of red blood cell in order to compensate for the low oxygen tension, which mimics chronic hypoxia. Such populations have haemoglobin levels of 1-2 g/dl higher than populations living closer to the sea level [48].

Problems may occur, when the body is unable to produce erythropoietin sufficiently in response to the oxygen condition. Under various pathological conditions including renal dysfunction, the erythropoietin production by the kidney is inhibited or its action in the bone marrow is reduced (haematological and solid tumours). Different factors may affect endogenous erythropoietin productions which are renal dysfunction, inflammation, infection, tumour growth, chemotherapy and bone marrow transplantation.

In the case of chronic kidney disease, progressive tubular damage and interstitial fibrosis results in a reduced ability of the kidney to produce erythropoietin. Different complex mechanisms may be responsible for the reduced erythropoietin production in patients with chronic kidney disease such as [49, 50]:
- Destruction of renal fibroblasts, which are responsible for the erythropoietin production
- Local inhibition of erythropoietin-production by inflammatory cytokines
- Missing compensation of erythropoietin production by the liver

Anaemia and disturbed erythropoietin production in patients with CKD occur mostly independently of the cause of renal insufficiency. There are, though, some exceptions, for example in patients with polycystic kidney disease, the endogenous erythropoietin plasma concentration is double as high as in other patients with CKD. Interstitial cells in the cystic wall are expressing the erythropoietin gene, but how cysts are stimulating the erythropoietin production remains unclear. CKD patients with hepatitis can also improve anaemia during infection, a fact which may be attributed to an increase of erythropoietin production in the liver [5].

Potential inhibitors of erythropoiesis

Erythroid cells of ureic patients still respond to recombinant erythropoietin treatment and the response of the bone marrow is not essentially reduced compared to healthy persons. Nevertheless, the erythropoiesis can be impaired by several factors:
- Inadequate dialysis: Increased dialysis may improve haemoglobin concentration in epoetin-naïve patients and patients treated with epoetin [51, 52].
- Deficiency of important co-factors (iron, folic acid) [53] and complications of renal insufficiency (hyperparathyroidism, aluminium intoxication) [54, 55] may reduce the response of the bone marrow to erythropoietin and lead to erythropoietin resistance. Resistance to erythropoietin is described in 1.7.
- Pro-inflammatory cytokines inhibit the endogenous erythropoietin production and the proliferation of erythroid progenitor cells in the bone marrow as well. In addition, they reduce the availability of iron [56].

Decreased red cell survival

Red cell survival decreases in response to the degree of renal insufficiency and progressing uraemia and may be reduced to a third of the normal value. In an experiment with uremic patients, it had been demonstrated that plasma factors of uremic patients must be responsible for the shortened red cell survival. Red cell survival was decreased in uremic patients receiving transfusions from healthy volunteers and in healthy volunteers receiving transfusions from uremic patients, red cell survival was in the normal range [57].

Disturbance of erythrocyte transport mechanism through the spleen may be another factor for reducing red cell survival [58]. The exact biochemical reasons for the shortened survival of red cells are still not fully understood.

Blood loss

Patients with chronic renal insufficiency loose regularly blood during haemodialysis and for laboratory tests. The estimated blood loss over thirty years ago was between 1- 4 litres a year [59]. The amount of blood loss may be reduced over time thanks to technical progress, yet it remains a relevant pathogenetic factor of renal anaemia. Nowadays, the blood loss is estimated at 2-10 ml per dialysis resulting in 300-1,500 ml of blood loss per year. For laboratory analysis, 200-300 ml of blood is taken, which correspond to 1,000-2,000 mg of iron loss per year. In peritoneal dialysis, blood loss is minor compared to haemodialysis. Another major source of external blood loss commonly associated with CKD is gastrointestinal bleeding and results not only in a decreased red cell concentration but also in a decreased iron concentration. It may essentially contribute to iron deficiency and, thereafter, hyporesponse to ESA-treatment in patients with CKD.

1.5 Clinical consequences of renal anaemia

The symptoms of anaemia in CKD patients are fatigue, depression and cognitive dysfunction. Anaemia leads to a decreased oxygen delivery to the tissues without reducing of the total oxygen consumption of the organism, which provokes acidosis and stimulates a compensatory mechanism as a response to the decreased oxygen delivery. Thus, peripheral vasodilatation occurs, stimulating the sympathetic activity. This induces renal vasodilatation with activation of the renin-angiotensin system and the release of antidiuretic hormone. The fluid retention probably leads to left ventricular growth and hypertrophy [31, 60]. In some patients, anaemia may provoke an increase in left ventricular mass, in other patients it also leads to cardiac dilatation. Myocardial remodelling increases the risk of arrhythmias, myocard infarction and sudden death. At the onset of the dialysis, many patients already have cardiovascular diseases such as cardiac failure (31%), angina pectoris (19%) and coronary artery disease (14%). A left ventricular hypertrophy occurs even in 74% of the patients at the start of dialysis [61]. Cardiovascular complications are the most common causes of death among patients on dialysis and occur approximately 10-20 times more frequently than those observed in the general population [61].

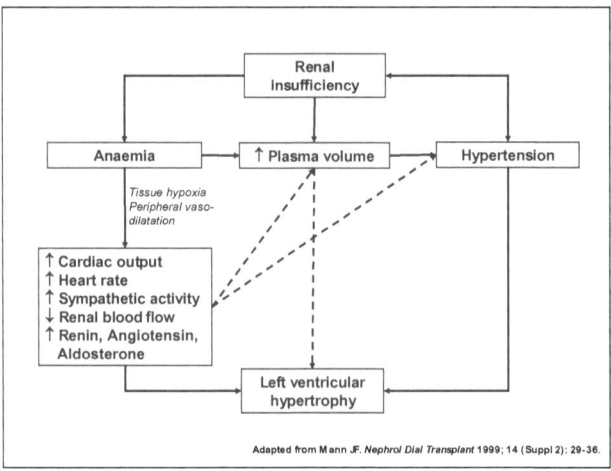

Figure 1-3: Clinical consequences of anaemia, adapted from Mann [60]

Several studies have demonstrated that anaemia is an independent risk factor for the development of left ventricular hypertrophy in dialysis patients. A decrease of the haemoglobin concentration of 1 g/dl was associated with a 42% increase of the risk of developing left ventricular hypertrophy and a 28% increase of the risk of developing of de novo congestive heart failure [62]. Several studies have shown that the lower the haemoglobin concentration, the greater the mortality on dialysis. Effective treatment of renal anaemia prevents cardiac damage, reduces cardiac mortality and improves the patients' well-being and is therefore crucial in the health care of patients with chronic kidney disease.

1.6 Anaemia treatment in ESRD

Before the introduction of recombinant human erythropoietin, patients with end-stage renal disease was regularly transfusion-dependent, which, as a consequence, lead to the formation of cytotoxic antibodies, iron overload and hepatitis. Today, three treatment options of erythropoiesis-stimulating agents (ESA) are available on the market for the treatment of renal anaemia, i.e. epoetin alfa (since 1988), epoetin beta (since 1990) and darbepoetin alfa (since 2001). Anaemia of CKD patients should be treated with ESAs if haemoglobin concentration consistently falls below 11 g/dl (haematocrit <33%) and all other causes of anaemia have been excluded.

In the following paragraph, the history of the identification of erythropoietin and the properties of the different ESAs are described in more detail.

1.6.1 Erythropoiesis-stimulating agents (ESA)

The identification, characterization and cloning of the human gene for erythropoietin made the causative therapy of renal anaemia possible. The concept of erythropoiesis was developed in the beginning of 1900 by Paul Carnot but it took more than 50 years to investigate this humoral mechanism and to find the production site of erythropoietin. In 1962, Goldwasser isolated erythropoietin for the first time from an anaemic sheep and later from anaemic patients. At that time, a tremendous quantity of urine from patients was necessary in order to isolate 70,000 U/mg. The cloning of EPO in 1985 and the subsequent availability of cloned DNA by using recombinant method made it possible to produce larger quantities of EPO protein [63, 64].

Recombinant human erythropoietin (rHuEPO)

Recombinant human erythropoietin is a glycoprotein which has approximately the same characteristics and molecular weight as the endogenous hormone. It consists of a 165-amino-acid protein chain, which is essential for the binding of the molecule to the receptor of the erythroid progenitor cells in the bone marrow. Four carbohydrate chains are connected to the protein by three N-glycolyzation and one O-glycolyzation site as depicted in Figure 1-4. The carbohydrate mojety of epoetin is approximately 40% with terminal sialic acids. Glycolyzation is important for the biological activity of EPO. Removal or modification of the glycan chains results in altered in vivo and in vitro activity. The number of sialic acid residues and the carbohydrate chains determine the pharmacodynamics, half-life and biologic activity of EPO [65, 66].

Recombinant human erythropoietin has been available as a drug since 1998 and is used in the clinical treatment of anaemia, especially anaemia caused by renal failure and by tumours. Epoetin alfa and epoetin beta are both synthesized in Chinese hamster ovary (CHO) cells. Recombinant erythropoietin is found to have small differences to the human serum EPO. The most prominent difference is the absence of tetra-sialyted oligosaccharide structure in the circulating EPO. In contrast, rHuEPO has relatively high content of tetra-sialyted oligosaccharide structures (epoetin alfa: 19%; epoetin beta: 46%), which are responsible for the increased half-life of glycoproteins and important with respect to in vivo and in vitro bioactivity of rHuEPO [67].

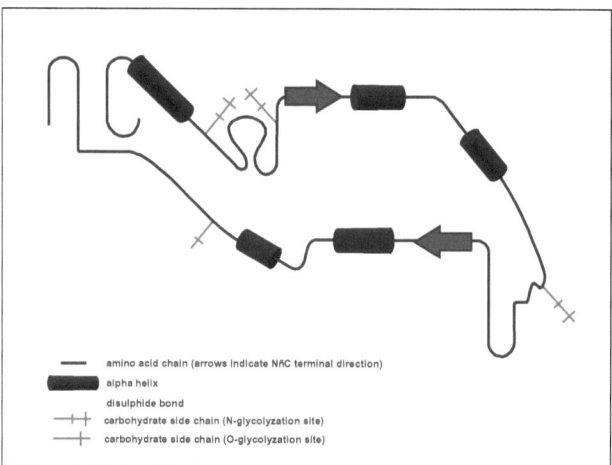

Figure 1-4: Molecule of rHuEPO

Variations in the glycolyzation and isoform between epoetin alfa and epoetin beta reveal differences in the pharmacokinetic and pharmacodynamic profile of these two molecules, whereas on the clinical level they are less important [67, 68]. The terminal elimination half-life of intravenous epoetin beta was 20% longer and the volume of distribution was significantly greater than observed with epoetin alfa. These differences between epoetin alfa and epoetin beta may be mainly explained by the different carbohydrate structure of the two molecules [69]. Table 1-3 provides an overview of the pharmacokinetic parameters of epoetin alfa and epoetin beta.

Darbepoetin alfa

Recently, a new generation of EPO replacement therapy was developed for the treatment of anaemia. Novel erythropoiesis stimulation protein (NESP) has a longer duration of action and therefore a longer half-life than rHuEPO. The increased serum half-life and longer duration of action compared to rHuEPO derive from its increased sialic acid content resulting from two additional carbohydrate chains [66]. Darbepoetin alfa has a 2-3 fold longer plasma half-life (see Table 1-3) [70], which allows prolonged dosing intervals. The recommended starting dose is 0.45 µg/kg administered 1x weekly either intravenously and subcutaneously. Darbepoetin may be administered every two weeks in patients stable on the 1x weekly dosing regimen and dosing interval may be prolonged up to 1 month [71]. A comparison of the molecules and physicochemical properties between rHuEPO and darbepoetin alfa can be seen in Table 1-3.

Value, mean ± SD or (range) where available	Epoetin beta[1]	Epoetin alfa[1]	Darbepoetin alfa (NESP)[2]
Half-life (h)	s.c. 24.2 ± 11.2 i.v. 8.9 ± 1.1*	s.c. 19.4 ± 10.7 i.v. 7.9 ± 1.0	s.c. 49 (27-89) i.v. 25.3
Clearance (ml/h/kg)	i.v. 7.9 ± 1.2	i.v. 8.2 ± 1.0	i.v. 1.85
Volume of distribution at steady state (Vss) (ml/kg)	i.v. 70.0 ± 10.4*	i.v. 63.8 ± 6.1	59.5
Time to maximum concentration (Tmax) (h)	s.c. 15 ± 7	s.c. 15 ± 8	s.c. 34
Bioavailability (%)	s.c. 32.7 ± 8.2	s.c. 31.9 ± 9.1	s.c. 36.9 (30-50)

[1] Adapted from Halstenson et al. [69]; [2] Adapted from SmPC of darbepoetin alfa [71]
*p<0.05 epoetin beta versus epoetin alfa

Table 1-3: Pharmacokinetic parameters of ESAs

1.6.2 Efficacy of ESAs

Dosing and route of administration

In this section, the efficacy of epoetin beta will be described in more detail, since the survey was performed with this substance. The efficacy of epoetin beta was investigated in a randomized, multicentre dose-finding study, where dialysis patients received 40 IU, 80 IU or 120 IU/kg three times a week intravenously. The dose of epoetin beta was then determined to be 40 IU/kg three times a week. Non-responding patients may receive increased doses step by step up to 720 IU/kg per week. When the target haematocrit was achieved, the dose of epoetin beta was reduced by 50%. The majority of the patients achieved a statistically significant increase in haematocrit with improved well-being and physical performance [72].

Subcutaneous administration of epoetin allows a dose reduction of 20-30% compared to the intravenous administration [73, 74], which is also reflected in the dosing recommenddation for subcutaneous administration of epoetin beta. The initial recommended dose of epoetin beta is for subcutaneous administraiton 20 IU/kg three times a week and for the intravenous administration 40 IU/kg three times a week [75]. These findings had been important to know in view to shift from intravenous to subcutaneous route of administration in haemodialysis patients in Europe, where approximately 50-60% of all dialysis patients received epoetin subcutaneously at the beginning of the survey "AIMS" [40].

The better efficacy of the subcutaneous administration of epoetin might be due to the longer terminal elimination half-life compared to the intravenous administration. Even though higher peak epoetin serum concentrations were achieved when administered intravenously, absolute reticulocyte response was far smaller than with the subcutaneous administration. Erythropoietic response is less related to the peak plasma concentration but more relevant to maintain a certain threshold concentration [69].

Administration frequency

The prolonged action of the subcutaneous administration of epoetin described in the pharmacokinetic investigations [69] and the first findings of the potential efficacy of the 1x weekly subcutaneous administration [76] were crucial for further investigations of the efficacy of epoetin beta at a reduced dosing frequency. Two large-scale studies of 1x weekly subcutaneous administration were performed in haemodialysis patients, which demonstrated that 1x weekly epoetin beta was as efficacious as a 2-3x weekly administration without significant increase in dose [77, 78]. The 1x weekly subcutaneous administration of epoetin was found to be efficacious not only in haemodialysis, but also in peritoneal dialysis [79] and pre-dialysis patients [80]. The study of Weiss et al. published in 1998 was the basis for the registration of the 1x weekly subcutaneous administration in stable patients with renal anaemia. The study included 158 stable haemodialysis patients on a 2-3x weekly dosing regimen with a haemoglobin level between 10 and 12.5 g/dl. The patients were randomized either to receive 1x weekly subcutaneous or to remain on their original regimen for 24 weeks. No significant differences were observed in haemoglobin levels and in weekly epoetin dose between both treatments, as can be seen in Table 1-4.

The European regulatory authority (EMEA = European Medicine Agency) approved the 1x weekly subcutaneous administration of epoetin beta in stable patients with renal anaemia at 17 September 2001. At that time, the preferred administration frequency of epoetin beta was 2-3x weekly in dialysis patients and there was only limited experience with a 1x weekly regimen. One of the objectives of the survey was to evaluate whether the 1x weekly regimen of epoetin beta was feasible and beneficial to dialysis patients in Switzerland. The survey also investigated the relevance of the 1x weekly subcutaneous administration in dialysis patients in Switzerland. In 2004, the regulatory authorities approved the administration of epoetin beta every two weeks in patients (s.c.) with renal anaemia who are stable on a 1x weekly subcutaneous treatment regimen.

Mean ± Standard devation (SD)	Group	Week 0	Week 6	Week 16	Week 24
Epoetin beta dose (IU/kg)	1x weekly	102 ± 17	107 ± 70	103 ± 68	106 ± 74
	control group	109 ± 49	112 ± 54	109 ± 57	115 ± 58
Haemoglobin (g/dl)	1x weekly	11.4 ± 0.6	11.1 ± 1.1	11.1 ± 1.1	11.1 ± 1.2
	control group	11.2 ± 0.6	11.3 ± 1.1	11.3 ± 0.9	11.2 ± 1.2

The changes between weeks 0-24 in the 1x weekly group and control group were not statistically significant,

Table 1-4: Efficacy of the 1x weekly subcutaneous administration of epoetin beta in stable haemodialysis patients

Table 1-5 provides an overview of the route of administration, patient type, dosing and dosing frequency. ESAs can be administered in haemodialysis, peritoneal dialysis, pre-dialysis and transplanted patients with renal anaemia with some exceptions for epoetin alfa. This is due to the contraindication of the subcutaneous administration of epoetin alfa in renal anaemia in Europe since 2002 (see 1.6.3). The subcutaneous administration of rHuEPO has greater efficacy than intravenous administration and allows dose savings of 20-30%. This difference between the subcutaneous and intravenous administration was not observed for darbepoetin alfa, even though half-life of the subcutaneous administration was prolonged as well.

Dosing frequency and route of administration	Epoetin beta [81]	Epoetin alfa [81]	Darbepoetin alfa (NESP) [81]
Route of administration	s.c. i.v.	i.v.	s.c. i.v.
Patient type	CKD, HD, PD, Tx	HD N/A for CKD, PD, Tx	CKD, HD, PD, Tx
Correction phase	s.c.: 3x 20 IU/kg/week i.v.: 3x 40 IU/kg/week	i.v.: 3x 50 IU/kg/week	s.c. or i.v.: 1x 0.45 µg/kg/week
Maintenance[1]	1x weekly s.c.[2] 1x /2 weeks s.c.[3] 3x weekly i.v.	3x weekly (i.v. only)	1x weekly s.c. or i.v. 1x /2 weeks s.c. or i.v.

[1] Dose reduction of 25-50% of the last dose administered in correction phase; [2] in stable patients with renal anaemia; [3] in stable renal anaemic patients on the 1x weekly s.c. administration of epoetin beta
N/A= not applicable because not licensed for use by this route [82]
CKD= chronic kidney disease patients, HD= haemodialysis, PD= peritoneal dialysis, Tx= transplantation

Table 1-5: Dosing frequency and route of administration of ESAs

1.6.3 Safety and tolerability of epoetin beta

The most common adverse events of epoetin beta are cardiovascular disease (20%), hypertension (17%), muscle cramps, headache, and pruritus. Hypertension was in most patients dose-dependent (17%) and declined in the second six months to 5% [75]. There was no significant increase in vascular access thrombosis or other thromboembolic events under the therapy of epoetin. Epoetin beta was well tolerated when administered subcutaneously [83]. The local pain at the injection site with subcutaneous administration was comparable to placebo and was significantly less frequent compared with epoetin alfa [77] or darbepoetin alfa [84]. The 1x weekly treatment regimen was also a well tolerated treatment regimen and comparable to the 2-3x weekly administration of epotin beta [77, 78].

An upsurge of antibody-mediated pure red-cell aplasia (PRCA) was observed in mainly one product, which resulted in the contraindication of the subcutaneous administration of epoetin alfa, outside US in 2002. No increase in the immunogenicity of epoetin beta had been observed and epoetin beta can still be administered subcutaneously and intravenously [85-87]. In Switzerland epoetin alfa and beta were predominately (approximately 70-80%) administered subcutaneously before 2002. A shift from the subcutaneous to the intravenous route of administration for epoetin beta was considered as well after the contraindication of the subcutaneous route of administration for epoetin beta. A change in the route of administration of epoetin beta was assessed in this survey, since the upsurge of pure red-cell aplasia occurred during the survey period.

1.6.4 Clinical benefits of the treatment with ESA

Treatment of renal anaemia with ESAs improves overall patient quality of life, physical, psychological and psychosocial aspects of everyday life. Studies also demonstrated a substantial improvement of exercise capacity and a better ability to perform physical activities [6, 11, 88-90].

Left ventricular hypertrophy is an independent risk factor for cardiac morbidity and mortality. Dialysis patients with a left ventricular hypertrophy (>165 g/m^2) had a 3.7-fold higher risk of death compared with patients without LVH [91]. Treatment with epoetin resulted in a substantial reduction of existing left ventricular hypertrophy in CKD patients [13, 32, 92]. Several studies have shown an association between the mortality on dialysis and haemoglobin. A decrease in haemoglobin of 1 g/dl was associated with a 14-18% increase in mortality [62, 93]. The treatment of anaemia with epoetin resulted in a 20% lower one-year overall mortality and in a 40% lower cardiovascular mortality in dialysis patients as compared to the control group, which did not receive epoetin [94, 95].

A relation between anaemia and mortality was also observed in the Lombardy Dialysis Registry [12] and in the study of Ma et al. [96]. Total mortality rate and the risk of hospitalization increased as the haematocrit level decreased in ESRD patients, which is illustrated in Figure 1-5. The lowest risk of death was observed in patients with a haematocrit level in the range of >32% and of 33-36%, respectively. Anaemia correction in dialysis patients resulted not only in a decreased mortality rate but also in a reduced hospitality rate. Patients with haematocrit levels lower than 30% had a 14-30% increased risk of hospitalization compared with patients in the control group showing a haematocrit level of 30-33%. The lowest risk for hospitalization was observed at a haematocrit level of 33-36% [97]. In a recent study of Li et al. hospitalization rate was lowest in patients with a haematocrit level of >36% [98].

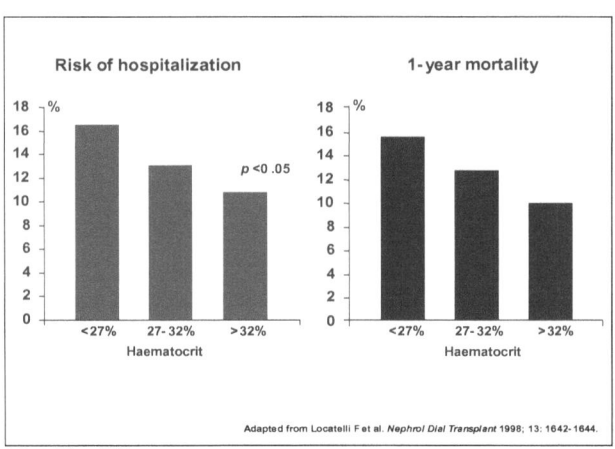

Adapted from [12]

Figure 1-5: Association between haematocrit and risk of hospitalization and mortality in ESRD patients.

The presence of anaemia during the early stage of chronic kidney disease may also lead to an acceleration of kidney damage. Several studies have demonstrated a beneficial effect on the progression of chronic kidney disease when treated with epoetin [99-101]. Early treatment of anaemia in patients with CKD showed to be beneficial by preventing cardiovascular complications and to slow down the decline of renal function.

1.7 Factors affecting response to ESAs

The revised European Best Practice Guidelines define ESAs as follow: "A resistance to ESAs should be suspected when a patient either fails to attain the target haemoglobin concentration while receiving more than 300 IU/kg/week (~20,000 IU/week) of epoetin or 1.5 µg/kg of darbepoetin alfa (~100 µg/week)" [82]. Instead of resistance, the term hyporesponsiveness is often used. The factors described in the following section may influence response to epoetin therapy.

Iron deficiency

The most common cause of hyporesponsiveness to ESAs is iron deficiency. Most dialysis patients under ESAs develop iron deficiency because of the continuous blood loss from gastrointestinal bleeding, blood drawing and haemodialysis (2 g iron per year) [102]. Adequate iron stores are important for achieving adequate response under ESA treatment, as illustrated in Figure 1-6.

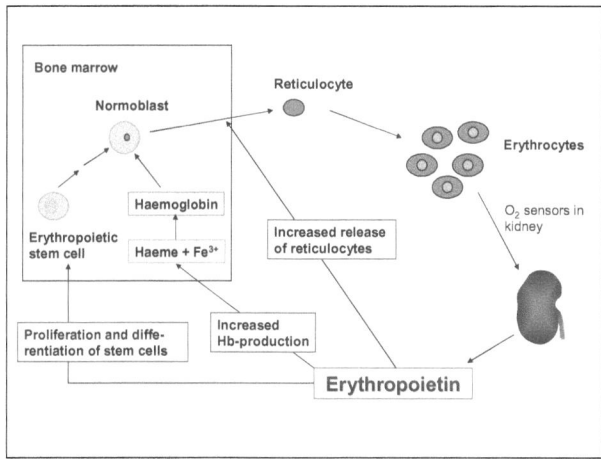

Figure 1-6: Iron and influence on erythropoietic response

European Best Practice Guidelines [40, 82] and the NKF-K/DOQI guidelines [103] recommend serum ferritin ≥100 µg/l, hypochromic red cells <10% or transferrin saturation of 20% in order to achieve and maintain target haemoglobin concentration of 11 g/dl in chronic kidney disease patients. Optimal supplementation consists of target serum ferritin of 200-500 µg/l and transferrin saturation of 30-40% (hypochromic red cells <2.5%) should be aimed in order to achieve these basic criteria. Absolute iron deficiency is likely to be present in patients with CKD when transferrin saturation (TSAT, TsF) falls below 20% and the serum ferritin concentration is less than 100 µg/l. Beside absolute iron deficiency, functional iron deficiency may occur in renal patients. Functional iron deficiency is characterized by the presence of adequate iron stores, but with the inability to sufficiently mobilize the iron in order to adequately support erythropoiesis. In this case, serum ferritin levels are normal, but transferrin saturation is normally below 20%.

Most dialysis patients require iron supplementation. Haemodialysis patients generally receive iron intravenously (25-100 mg/week) and peritoneal dialysis patients rather orally. Iron supplementation should be administered cautiously in patients with excessive iron stores, i.e. with serum ferritin concentrations above 500 µg/l [104, 105]. Likewise, the guidelines recommend a threshold level above which additional iron should generally not be given (800 µg/l and/or transferrin saturation > 50%) [82, 103]. Table 1-6 provides an overview of the target iron levels in chronic kidney disease patients recommended by the EBPG [40, 82].

Recommended iron supplementation in CKD patients [82]	Optimal	Adequate	Deficiency
Serum ferritin (µg/l)	200-500	100	<100
Transferrin saturation (%)	30-40	>20	<20
Hypochromic red cells (%)	<2.5	<10	>10

Table 1-6: Recommendations of iron targets for anaemia treatment in CKD according to the EBPG

Infection, inflammation and concomitant diseases

Infection and inflammation may influence epoetin response mediated by inflammatory cytokine such as tumour necrosis factor (TNF) and interleukin-1. An elevated C-reactive protein level is often associated with inflammation and/or infection and may be a predictor of resistance to ESAs [106]. In the case of hyperparathyroidism, especially in the presence of osteitis fibrosa, higher epoetin doses are generally required since bone marrow is infiltrated with fibrosis [54].

Multiple myeloma patients may respond to treatment with ESA but they usually require higher doses. Patients with malignancies generally respond less to ESA therapies. Inflammations and malignancies reduce iron availability for erythropoiesis. Inflammatory factors such as interleukins and TNF are involved and reduce proliferation of the precursor cells and therefore the efficacy of ESAs [39, 107, 108].

Other factors

There were controversial findings about the influence of angiotensin-converting enzyme inhibitors (ACE inhibitors) concerning the response to ESA. Some reports suggest that there is an inhibition of ESA by ACE inhibitorsI [109, 110] and others demonstrated that there is no association between the dose of ESAs and ACE inhibitor therapy [111, 112]. In the case of hyporesponsiveness to ESA therapy, EBPG recommend, especially when high dose of ACE inhibitor are used, to take into consideration a treatment stop of ACE inhibitor therapy and to evaluate treatment response in its absence [40]. AT_1-receptor antagonists seem to have no proven influence on ESA response even though reports confirming were registered [113, 114]. Other factors influencing response to ESA are folic acid and vitamin B_{12} deficiencies which have to be observed with increasing ESA dose requirements in dialysis patients [40].

In the present "AIMS" survey, hyporesponsiveness to epoetin beta treatment was assessed with respect to the iron status, since iron deficiency is the main cause of resistance to ESAs in dialysis patients. Furthermore the relationship between epoetin beta-dose and achieved haemoglobin level was investigated in more detail.

1.8 Target haemoglobin level

EBPG [40] and the NKF-K/DOQI guidelines [15] recommend initiating ESA-terhapy when the haemoglobin level falls below 11 g/dl. European Best Practice Guidelines (EBPG) recommend to maintain a target haemoglobin concentration in patients with chronic kidney disease of >11 g/dl (haematocrit >33%), which should not exceed 14 g/dl [40, 82]. Haemoglobin concentration above 12 g/dl is not recommended for patients with severe cardiovascular diseases unless symptoms occur, for patients with diabetes and peripheral vascular disease, for reasons of increased risk of thrombosis. However, patients with chronic pulmonary disease may benefit from a higher target haemoglobin level [40, 82]. The upper limit for haemoglobin level is not clearly defined by the EBPG.

Ideally, the target haemoglobin concentration in patients with CKD, including end-stage renal disease (ESRD) treated with any erythropoietic agent would be defined as the value that is clinically optimal for each patient, based upon their individual circumstances, such as general level of function, employment, co-morbidities (ischemic coronary disease, heart failure). Up to now, there is a lack of data on which to base such individual treatment decisions. Furthermore, optimal target haemoglobin level to aim at in CKD patients is still unclear and remains to be defined. There is evidence that better outcomes were associated with higher haemoglobin levels (between 11-12 g/dl) than with haemoglobin levels below this range. Support for partial or full normalization of haemoglobin concentration is less consistent. The study of Ma et al. demonstrated a progressive increase in the risk of all-cause and cardiac death in patients with haematocrit levels below the range of 33-36%. The mortality and hospitalization rate was not lower in patients at a haematocrit level of >36% [12, 96, 98]. Moreover, the US Normal Haematocrit Study showed rather unexpected adverse outcome, suggesting a potential increase of mortality and morbidity risk with normal haemoglobin levels [115]. However, in a recent study of Li et al. the hospitalization rate was reduced at that very haemoglobin level [98].

At present, guidelines based on clinical evidence support maintaining haemoglobin levels at the range of 11-12 g/dl for patients with chronic kidney disease. Quality of life may be improved at normalized haemoglobin levels, however, there is not yet convincing evidence to support normalization of haemoglobin levels in CKD patients since cardiovascular morbidity and mortality did not improve at that level. Increasing target haemoglobin concentration would also have a significant impact on costs. Two large studies which are currently conducted will provide more information concerning the value and benefits of haemoglobin level normalization [116, 117].

1.9 Summary and rationales

Nearly 90% of chronic kidney disease patients with a glomerular filtration rate (GFR) of less than 25-30 ml/min have anaemia, many of them with haemoglobin levels below 10 g/dl [2]. The treatment of renal anaemia was revolutionized by the introduction of recombinant human erythropoietin more than 15 years ago. The treatment with erythropoietic agents (ESAs) allows a causal therapy of renal anaemia and is nowadays a well-established therapy. Today, most patients on dialysis, either peritoneal dialysis or haemodialysis, and with presence of anaemia receive treatment with ESAs. The process of defining optimal dosage regimens and optimal target haemoglobin levels requires more time and scientific discussions about target haemoglobin and individualized treatment strategies are still ongoing. Guidelines for the treatment of renal anaemia were first issued in 1996 by the US National Kidney Foundation Dialysis Outcome Quality Initiative (NKF-DOQI) and in 1998, representatives of the ERA-EDTA and the societies of nephrology of the European Union, Central and Eastern European countries established the European Best Practice Guidelines for the management of anaemia in patients with chronic renal failure (EBPG). For the first time, recommendations for the treatment of renal anaemia were offered, with the objective to improve clinical practice and to provide evidence-based standards for the treatment of anaemia in CKD patients. Target haemoglobin level in renal anaemia therapy was defined to be >11 g/dl for patients with chronic kidney disease and for patients with cardiovascular diseases or diabetes a haemoglobin level of 11-12 g/dl should be aimed at. Revised EBPG (issued in May 2004) recommend a target haemoglobin level of >11g/dl, which should be defined for individual patients, taking gender, age, activity and co-morbid conditions into account [82].

Two surveys were performed after the initiation of the EBPG, the End-stage Renal Disease (ESRD) Core Indicator Project and the European Survey in Anaemia Management (ESAM), in order to evaluate the implementation of the guidelines [118, 119]. The findings suggest that a high proportion of dialysis patients (47% of haemodialysis and 40% of peritoneal dialysis patients [119]) did not achieve the moderate target haemoglobin level of 11 g/dl recommended by the guidelines. This might be explainable by a number of historical and economic reasons. In earlier treatments studies, haemoglobin concentrations between 10 and 11 g/dl were aimed at, which were considered as appropriate target haemoglobin concentrations, and which became the standard practice in most dialysis centres.

Currently, partial correction of anaemia is aspired in chronic kidney disease patients; however, recent studies indicated a link between suboptimal haemoglobin concentrations and cardiovascular disease with CKD [91, 120, 121]. In contrast, the US Normal Hematocrit Study, which was designed to investigate the risks and benefits of higher target haematocrit levels (42%) compared to lower targets in haemodialysis patients. Unexpectedly, a higher incidence of death was found in the group with higher haematocrit concentrations, which resulted in the conclusion that haemoglobin normalization can not be recommended in haemodialysis patients [115].

The Guidelines call for regular re-evaluation and that the impact of the guidelines on clinical practice be re-investigated subsequently. The 12-month practice based, open-intervention survey *Anaemia Management in dialysis patients in Switzerland* "AIMS" reflects this requirement; it evaluated current treatment practices in renal anaemia in order to reveal new insights into renal anaemia management in Switzerland. It was the first survey performed in Switzerland which ascertained long-term data of current anaemia management in dialysis patients after the edition of the EBPG. The survey "AIMS" further assessed the adherence of current anaemia management in Swiss dialysis centres to the European Best Practice Guidelines and potential deviations. The specific aim was to characterize the use of epoetin beta, specifically the dosing frequency (1x *vs* 2–3x weekly) and the route of administration (i.v. vs s.c.). Additionally, it assessed physicians' haemoglobin target levels in dialysis patients and whether they were adapted according to the patients' co-morbidity stage.

It may be more appropriate to individualize anaemia treatment in CKD patients and to adapt target haemoglobin levels according to the physical conditions of each patient. This, however, requires further clinical trials defining different target haemoglobin levels for well-defined patient groups and new guidelines for the treatment of anaemia in CKD.

2. Objectives

The present survey *AnaemIa Management in dialysis patients in Switzerland* "AIMS", was one of the first surveys conducted in the post-EBPG (European Best Practice Guidelines for the management of anaemia in patients with chronic renal failure) era in Switzerland. The objectives of "AIMS" were to provide long-term data from Swiss dialysis centres on current anaemia management and to assess the quality of anaemia control in comparison to the current guidelines [40]. The specific objectives of this practice-based, open-intervention survey are the following:

1. **AnaemIa Management in dialysis patients in Switzerland "AIMS".**
   Assess the quality of anaemia control achieved with epoetin beta in dialysis patients in Switzerland.
2. **Adherence of anaemia management in dialysis patients in Switzerland to current guidelines (EBPG).**
   Assess Swiss anaemia management in dialysis patients and physicians' targets in anaemia treatment. Compare current anaemia treatment with the European Best Practice Guidelines (EBPG) for the management of anaemia in patients with chronic renal failure.
3. **Efficacy and safety of anaemia management with epoetin beta.**
   Assess the relevance of the 1x weekly administration of epoetin beta in dialysis patients in Switzerland. Compare two dosing schedules of epoetin beta and assess the efficacy and safety of epoetin beta.
4. **Individualizing anaemia management in dialysis patients in Switzerland – Do co-morbidities and patients' health influence physicians' target haemoglobin level?**
   Assess the prevalence of diagnosis and co-morbidities in dialysis patients in Switzerland and compare it to the findings of international registries. Assess whether physicians individualize target haemoglobin levels according to the patients' clinical condition (co-morbidities, diagnosis).

3. Methods and baseline characteristics

3.1 Objectives and design

Anaemla Management in dialysis patients in Switzerland "AIMS" was a practice-based, open-intervention survey conducted in different Swiss dialysis centres with the purpose to evaluate current anaemia management. It was a prospective, open-label, non-randomized survey initiated in June 2002. Patient recruitment was planned to be finished one year later, in June 2003, and was extended until December 2003. The observation period lasted 12 months. Study interruption was possible at any time during the survey. The primary objective of the survey was to assess anaemia management with epoetin beta in dialysis patients in Switzerland. Efficacy of epoetin beta, route of administration, dosing frequency and weekly dose of epoetin beta were therefore assessed. As to the second objective, individual targets of anaemia management were investigated and current anaemia treatment was compared with the current guidelines. The third objective was to examine the relevance of the 1x weekly administration of epoetin beta and to compare the efficacy and safety of two dosing schedules of epoetin beta. Finally, the prevalence of co-morbidities in dialysis patients in Switzerland and its impact on physicians' treatment behaviour in anaemia were assessed.

Practice-based survey

Practice-based surveys are clinical reports of the medical practice with the purpose to collect data of the current therapeutically applied medical treatment without interference of a third party and can only be performed within registered indications, dosages and formulations. Swiss legislation allows for systematic clinical reports so-called "Praxiserfahrungsberichte" (PEB) (Rapport d'expérience pratique [REP]). In such surveys, data on licenced and approved drugs and formulations can be collected with no approval of ethical committees. In the Swissmedic Bulletin (3/2000), "Praxiserfahrungsberichte" were defined as follows [122]:

"*Praxiserfahrungsberichte sind Berichte aus der ärztlichen Praxis zuhanden einer pharmazeutischen Firma. Dabei geht es um Sammeln und Erfassen von Daten bei der durch Dritte unbeeinflussten und therapeutisch üblichen Anwendung von Heilmitteln, welche bei der Swissmedic registriert sind. Solche Berichte beziehen sich auf die von der Swissmedic zugelassenen Indikationen, Dosierungen und galenischen Formen.*"

In contrast to clinical studies, the administration of a medical product within practice-based surveys is an open intervention and not designated by a study protocol. Interference in treatment strategies and requirements for additional medical analysis exceeding medical routine need the approval from the ethical committee and from the authorities (Swissmedic).

The main objectives of the survey were to evaluate current anaemia treatment in Swiss dialysis centres and, secondly, to evaluate the importance of the 1x weekly dosing regimen of epoetin beta in Swiss dialysis centres. No randomized clinical trial is needed for this scope, and reliable data can be obtained within a survey. Generally, surveys are less time-consuming and less complicated to perform, which may encourage more dialysis centres to participate. Surveys may provide certain risks of bias but they generally reflect the real everyday situation better than clinical trials. Representativity and risk of bias are discussed in section 3.8, page 46.

3.2 Sampling method

In order to make a reliable generalization about certain characteristics, the sample has to represent the population in terms of these characteristics. One approach to ensure a representative sample of the dialysis patients in Switzerland is to choose the sample randomly out of the totally 2,483 dialysis patients treated in 70 dialysis centres (source: SVK [Schweizerischer Verband für Gemeinschaftsaufgaben der Krankenversicherer] as of 31.12.2002) [22]. In our health care system, patients are not directly accessible and can not be randomly selected.

For this reason, dialysis centres have to be contacted in order to include dialysis patients. Certain criteria should be taken into consideration in view of the selection of dialysis centres, since the findings of our survey should reflect country-wide practice of anaemia management in dialysis patients. The best method to gain a random sample of dialysis centres would be either to cluster samples or to sample at equal intervals (f. ex. inclusion of every third patient). These procedures are, however, not practicable in the scope of such surveys since they are performed on a voluntary basis, and it was also expected that randomly selected dialysis centres would not agree to participate. We further analysed the dialysis centres in terms of their geographical distribution and their structure (size, hospital, non-hospital, public or private) in order to make a reasonable selection. Two third of all dialysis centres are located in the Swiss German part (47), 19 in the Swiss French part and 4 in the Swiss Italien part. Most dialysis centres are located in hospitals, and a minority (23%) are private dialysis centres. Nevertheless, the great majority of dialysis patients are treated in hospitals, but we decided to include patients of private dialysis centres as well. For, it could be argued that multi-morbid patients are more likely to be treated at universities or bigger hospitals and that patients in better clinical conditions are in private dialysis centres. This made us to contact all dialysis centres in Switzerland in order to achieve a higher participation rate and inclusion of patients from different dialysis centres all over the country.

The recruitment was initiated in June 2002 and was on a volontary basis (no random sample). The survey was presented to the responsible nephrologist of each dialysis centre. Participating dialysis centres were asked to include as many dialysis patients of their centre as possible in order to minimize a potential selection bias. Representativity of the patients included in "AIMS" is discussed in section 3.7.

After positive consent of the dialysis centres, they were provided with report forms for each patient designated for survey inclusion. The target population comprised adult patients undergoing regular haemodialysis or peritoneal dialysis. Patients were screened by the investigators according to their medical history and were allowed to be included when fulfilling the eligibility criteria. The inclusion and exclusion criteria were defined as follows:

Inclusion criteria
- Adult dialyzed patients (haemodialysis or peritoneal dialysis; ≥ 18 years old)
- Epoetin-naïve patients with newly diagnosed renal anaemia
- Dialysis patients on ongoing epoetin therapy
- Adequate iron status: Ferritin ≥ 200 µg/l, transferrin saturation $\geq 20\%$
- Adequate dialysis quality (Kt/V ≥ 1.2)
- No minimal time on dialysis was requested

Exclusion criteria
- Unstable angina pectoris
- Untreated hypertension
- Haemoglobinopathy
- Haemolysis
- Gastrointestinal bleeding
- Acute infection or unstable systemic inflammatory disease
- Epilepsy
- Pregnancy
- Lactation
- Deficiency of vitamin B_{12} (<200 ng/l)
- Deficiency of ferritin (<200 µg/l)
- Deficiency of folic acid (<2 µg/l)
- Planned surgery during the survey period (except fistula surgery)
- Known hypersensitivity to epoetin beta

All patients fulfilling the eligibility criteria according to the investigator were allowed to be included in the survey.

3.3 Sample size

The participation rate was estimated to be 10-20%. Consequently, we estimated a participation of approximately 150-200 patients, representing 6-8% of the total dialysis population in Switzerland, based on the source of SVK (as of 31.12.2002) [22].

Different analyses were planned to be performed in order to detect differences between treatment groups (for example to compare the efficacy of the 1x weekly administration to the 2-3x weekly dosing regimen of epoetin beta). A sample size calculation was performed using the formula below. A sample size of 146 (72.4 patients per group) was computed in order to achieve a 90% power to detect a difference in mean haemoglobin of 0.6 g/dl between the two groups with a known standard deviation of 1.0 g/dl and a significance level (alpha) of 0.05 (confidence interval of 95%) using a two-sided two-sample t-test.

$$N = \frac{2\sigma^2 \left[\Phi^{-1}(1-\alpha) - \Phi^{-1}(\beta)\right]^2}{(\mu_1 - \mu_2)^2}$$

$\Phi(x)$ = Area under the standard normal curve from $-\infty$ to x
α = type-1 error; β = type-2 error

Assuming that up to 20% of patients would not be eligible for the analysis, 180 patients (90 patients per group) were the requested sample size in order to detect differences of 0.6 g/dl with a confidence interval of 95%.

3.4 Treatment recommendations and concomitant medications

Dosing regimen of epoetin beta

Epoetin beta can be administered subcutaneously or intravenously depending on the clinical practice at the respective dialysis centre. With regard to individual dose selection, the dosage recommended by the specific product characteristics (SmPC) of epoetin beta should be followed [81, 123] and/or the European Best Practice Guidelines for the management of anaemia in patients with chronic renal failure [40] should be considered.

Prescribing information of epoetin beta: Correction phase: The recommended dosage for subcutaneous administration is 3x 20 IU/kg/week and for intravenous administration 3x 40 IU/kg/week. The epoetin dose may be doubled after four weeks if haematocrit increase was smaller than 0.5% per week. Further dose increments of 3x 20 IU/kg/week are allowed if necessary. Maintenance phase: The last administered epoetin dose can be reduced by 50%. In case of subcutaneous administration, the weekly dose can be given as an injection 1x per week and stable patients on a 1x weekly regimen can be switched to 1x every two weeks administration. The maximum doses should not exceed 720 IU/kg/week [75, 81].

European Best Practice Guidelines: Initial epoetin administration [40]: The starting dose of epoetin should be 50-150 IU/kg/week (4,000-8,000 IU/week), administered 2-3x a week. For intravenous administration, the starting dose should be in the upper range (typically 6,000 IU/week) three times a week. If the increase of haemoglobin concentration was <1 g/dl over a 4 week period, the dose of epoetin should be increased by 25%. If the increase of Hb level was >2.5 g/dl or exceed the target Hb concentration, the weekly dose of epoetin should be reduced by 25-50%. Recommended target haemoglobin level is ≥11 g/dl in chronic renal failure patients.

Iron supplementation and concomitant medication

Iron deficiency may cause a reduced erythropoietic response to epoetin therapy. For this reason, iron status measurements were recommended to be performed throughout the survey. This should include serum ferritin concentration and transferrin saturation, if performed during the survey. The following cut-off levels were defined as iron deficiency according to the EBPG: Serum ferritin <100 μg/l and transferrin saturation <20%. All patients included in the survey should be iron-repleted. For patients on dialysis, serum ferritin levels between 200-500μg/l and transferrin saturation of 30-40% are as optimum levels recommended. Iron supplementation should be followed according to the EBPG [40, 82].

All medications and treatments for renal anaemia and other concomitant diseases were permitted.

3.5 Survey methodology and data collection

AnaemIa Management of dialysis patients in Switzerland "AIMS" (objective 1)

The first objective was to assess anaemia treatment of dialysis patients cared in Swiss dialysis centres. Clinical report forms (CRFs), tailored to this first objective were prepared. The pre-printed data report forms consisted of an information form for physicians defining survey aim, inclusion and exclusion criteria, survey duration and procedure, and a flow chart showing summarizing the survey proceedings. Furthermore, it contained a patient registration form, a monthly patient report form, a final report for survey end or interruption and a spontaneous adverse event report form.

At patient registration the collected data included the following assessments:
- Aetiology of chronic renal failure, concomitant diseases, selected dialysis treatment modalities, dry weight and age were registered. The questionnaire contained pre-selections of potential diagnosis and concomitant diseases of chronic kidney disease (CKD) similar to multiple choice questionnaires. The most common diagnoses were already listed in the questionnaire, which were diabetic nephropathy, glomerulonephritis, pyelonephritis/interstitial nephritis and others.

The following selection of diagnosis was given: coronary artery disease, heart failure, diabetes, hypertension, and others. The section "others" concerned the option to specify and/or to add further diagnosis and concomitant diseases which were not listed.
- Laboratory parameters at baseline: haemoglobin at patient registration, and, if available, serum ferritin, transferrin saturation, serum creatinine were registered.
- Anaemia treatment at baseline and anaemia pre-treatment was documented at patient registration, including dosage, frequency, route of administration of epoetin beta and other anti-anaemic medications.

After patient registration, anaemia treatment and the quality of the anaemia management were assessed monthly for an observation period of 12 months. Physicians were asked to document monthly the following laboratory parameters and anaemia treatments:
- Laboratory parameter: haemoglobin (g/dl), serum ferritin*, transferrin saturation* and serum creatinine* (*if measured)
- Current anaemia treatment: dose, administration frequency and route of administration of epoetin beta and other anti-anaemic medications.

Laboratory parameters were documented if performed in the course of the clinical routine. No additional laboratory parameters exceeding the medical routine were requested to be performed.

Adverse events in relation to the epoetin beta treatment were requested to be documented in a separate spontaneous adverse event form. Reported serious adverse events had to be addressed to Swissmedic within 15 days at the latest and spontaneous non-serious adverse events within 60 days, according to the "Arzneimittelverordnung (Art. 35, 36)". A serious adverse event is defined as any experience that suggests a significant hazard, contraindication, side effect or precaution. A serious adverse event occurs if the event
- is fatal (result in death)
- is life-threatening
- required in-patient hospitalization or prolongation of existing hospitalization
- resulted in persistent or significant disability/incapacity
- is a congenital anomaly birth defect
- is medically significant or requires intervention to prevent one of or another than the outcomes listed above.

The monthly documentations of each patient were reported every three months after survey initiation. At survey end or interruption (drop-out, death or other reasons), the final report form needed to be completed by stating the reasons for survey discontinuation (other medication, transplantation, other reasons) and the clinical benefits of the epoetin beta treatment.

The scheme provides an overview of the schedule of assessments (see Table 3-1).

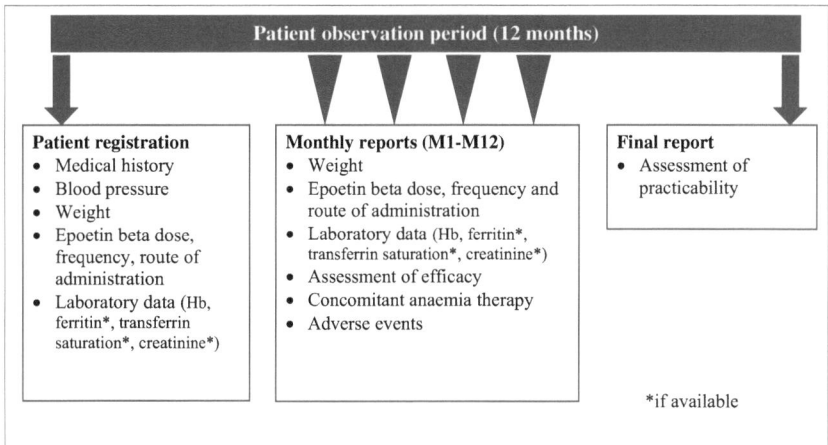

Table 3-1: Flow chart of assessments

All Swiss dialysis centres were contacted for survey participation. 28 of totally 70 Swiss dialysis centres participated in the survey. The received filled-in data report forms were examined on completeness of mandatory data and validated prior to data entry. Mandatory data were previously defined on the information sheet for physicians. Non-mandatory data were marked in the report forms and asked to fill in if available. Centres were contacted for missing mandatory data and requested to complete forms with missing data. Data were defined as mandatory for patient's dry weight, haemoglobin, dosage, route of administration and frequency of epoetin treatment. Some of the non-mandatory data were not available for all 340 patients (=shown in analysis as unknown or missing). All analyses were performed in all 340 eligible patients. All data of the report forms were entered in an excel database.

Adherence of Anaemia management in dialysis patients in Switzerland to current guidelines (EBPG) (objective 2)

A questionnaire was sent to all participating centres with the purpose to assess physicians' targets for anaemia management. Participating nephrologists were asked to provide target aims for haemoglobin, serum ferritin and transferrin saturation in dialysis patients at their dialysis centre. For the questionnaire see Appendix II. Anaemia management and centre-specific targets in Swiss dialysis centres were compared to current guidelines by using the European Best Practice Guidelines and the recently published revised European Best Practice Guidelines for the management of anaemia in patients with chronic renal failure (EBPG) [40, 82].

Efficacy and safety of anaemia management with epoetin beta (objective 3)

In this analysis, the relevance and the efficacy of the 1x weekly administration of epoetin beta was assessed. Subgroup-analyses were performed comparing the efficacy of the 1x administration with the 2-3x weekly administration of epoetin beta. The primary efficacy parameters of the analysis were area under the curve (AUC) for haemoglobin and for mean weekly epoetin beta dose per kilogram body weight. Secondary outcome parameters were mean haemoglobin concentrations and mean weekly epoetin dose per kilogram body weight as well as changes in haemoglobin from baseline. Furthermore, it was evaluated if the 1x weekly dosing regimen of epoetin beta was feasible and beneficial to dialysis patients in Switzerland. Safety parameters were adverse events occurring during the survey and mortality. We are aware that subgroup analyses of the kind are prone to bias; nevertheless, they reveal information about the relevance and feasibility of the 1x weekly administration of epoetin beta in the clinical practice of Swiss dialysis centres.

Individualizing anaemia management – Influence of co-morbidities on physicians' target haemoglobin (objective 4)

The prevalence of diagnosis and co-morbidities of dialysis patients included in "AIMS" were compared to the US and European registry (USRDS and ERA-EDTA registry). We further analysed whether anaemia treatment was adapted in respect of the clinical condition of each patients and whether co-morbidities had an influence on anaemia treatment. These informations were gathered on a separate questionnaire assessing physicians' target haemoglobin level in respect of the patients' co-morbid condition. All participating dialysis centres were asked to fill in this questionnaire.

3.6 Statistical analysis

Demographical and efficacy analysis

All data deriving from the questionnaires were entered in an excel database. Simple statistics was performed with Excel 2002 and complex statistical analysis with SAS statistical program version 8.2 (SAS, Institute, Cary, NC, USA) or the Epi-Info®, version 3.2. All patients fulfilling the exclusion and inclusion criteria (section 3.2, page 37) and who received at least one treatment of epoetin beta were included in the statistical analysis. Missing values of haemoglobin, body weight, epoetin dosage, frequency, serum ferritin and transferrin saturation were replaced by using the last observation carried forward (LOCF) method. The last visit was defined as the last observation carried forward. Data were checked for completeness. Drop-out patients (see 3.8.1, page 46) were eliminated before running the calculation. Demographic and baseline data are summarized by means and median of descriptive statistics. Point prevalence was calculated for diagnosis and co-morbidities of the included dialyses patients at patient registration (=baseline). All prevalence data are unadjusted data for age and gender. All statistical tests were two-sided and significance was proved on a 0.05 p-level.

Standard descriptive statistics (mean, standard deviation, confidence interval) were calculated for all study variables including haemoglobin, epoetin dosage, administration frequency, route of administration, serum ferritin and transferrin saturation. Categorical variables were presented in absolute number and percentage. The χ^2-test was used for the comparison of categorical variables. Continuous variables were compared using the Students' t-test, Wilcoxon two-sample and Kruskal-Wallis test where appropriate. Correlations were performed by using the Kendall Tau test or by using a simple linear regression analysis of Excel 2002. A longitudinal analysis for efficacy parameters (epoetin dosage and haemoglobin) was performed on a monthly base unless significant deviations from the time schedule occurred. In this case the data were assigned to the specified time interval. Univariate and multivariate regression was performed in order to assess the influence of diagnosis and co-morbidities on treatment response to epoetin beta.

Subgroup analysis of primary variables

A subgroup analysis was performed in order to assess the efficacy of the 1x weekly administration compared to the 2-3x weekly administration of epoetin beta in dialysis patients included in "AIMS". Haemoglobin over time and epoetin dose over time were the relevant parameters for the efficacy comparison of the two dosing regimens. The area under the curve (AUC) was calculated for those parameters. The AUC for haemoglobin was calculated for 6 months (baseline, month 1-6) using the following formula:

$$\text{AUC Hb} = \sum_{i=1}^{6} \frac{\text{Hb [Visit i]} + \text{Hb [Visit i-1]}}{2} * 30 \text{ days}$$

The second primary variable for the subgroup analysis was the epoetin dose per kg body weight. The body weight was measured every month after dialysis session (dry weight). The AUC was calculated for the weekly epoetin dose for 6 months using the following formula:

$$\text{AUC Dose} = \sum_{i=1}^{6} \frac{\text{dose [Visit i]} + \text{dose [Visit i-1]}}{2} * 30 \text{ days}$$

Confidence intervals were used to compare the efficacy of the two treatment regimens. For haemoglobin values the difference between means and the 95% confidence intervals was calculated. The 1x weekly regimen can be considered as therapeutically comparable if the confidence interval of the 1x weekly group lies within the range ±0.5 g/dl of the reference interval of the 2-3x weekly group. For the epoetin dose the difference between the average doses in both treatment groups was not expected to be higher than 10%. T-test and Wilcoxon-ranking test were performed to examine group differences in epoetin dose, serum ferritin concentrations and transferrin saturation.

Safety variables

All patients who received at least one dose of epoetin beta after patient registration were included in the safety analysis. The safety population corresponded to the treatment population. All reported adverse events occurring during observation had to be documented in the spontaneous adverse event form and sent to the authority (Swissmedic) or to the Drug Safety department of the manufacturer. Death or other serious adverse events related to the study medication were requested to be reported within 15 days to the authority (Swissmedic) or to the manufacturer. Deaths of patients not related to the study medication were reported in the final report form. Kaplan-Meier method was used to plot survival and mortality curves.

3.7 Representativity of the "AIMS" survey

As previously described, the population included in "AIMS" was not a random sample, although all dialysis centres were contacted. This is due to the fact that the participation was on a voluntary basis and not all contacted dialysis centres agreed to participate. This makes the question rise about the representativity of the sample. If the sample does not represent the respective population, it is termed biased [124] and the findings allow only conclusions about the sample itself and not for the respective population. Therefore, it is crucial to make sure that the included patients are a representative sample of the dialysis population in Switzerland.

Selected dialysis centres in Switzerland were characterized in terms of size, structure (public or private hospital, private centres) and geographical distribution in order to assess potential differences between the participating centres and those not participating. These data provide important information regarding the representativity of our sample. The structures of the Swiss dialysis centres are shown in Table 3-2. 77% of all dialysis centres in Switzerland are located in hospitals, whereof 5 are at university, 44 at regional hospitals and 5 are private hospitals. 23% of the dialysis centres (n=16) are private centres. The proportion of dialysis centres deriving from hospitals and private centres in the "AIMS" survey corresponded to the overall situation of dialysis centres in Switzerland (see Table 3-2). In our survey, 3 of 5 university hospitals, 16 of 44 regional hospitals, 3 of 5 private hospital and 4 of 16 private dialysis centres participated. No differences were detected between the participating centres and those not participating in respect of size and structure (public hospital, private hospital, and private dialysis centre), although more dialysis centres from the French speaking part participated. Nevertheless, the participating centres were representative for all dialysis centres in Switzerland.

Structure of dialysis centres	University hospitals n (%)	Regional hospitals n (%)	Private hospitals n (%)	Private dialysis centres n (%)
Total number of dialysis centres (n=70)	5 (7.1)	44 (62.9)	5 (7.1)	16 (22.9)
Centres participating in the survey (n=26)	3 (11.5)	16 (61.6)	3 (11.5)	4 (15.4)

Table 3-2: Structure of dialysis centres in Switzerland and in "AIMS"

It is also important that the selected dialysis patients were representative. A potential selection bias could be reduced if a high proportion of patients per dialysis centre were included (cluster sample). The great majority of the included dialysis patients were pre-treated with epoetin beta (80%), which increased the representativity of them. Therefore, the proportion of included patients (pre-treated with epoetin beta) and of the total number of patients treated with epoetin beta was analysed per dialysis centre (source: data of the SVK, as of 31.12.2002) [125].

Figure 3-1 provides an overview of this analysis. 10 dialysis centres included more than 80% and 15 centres more than 60% of all patients treated with epoetin beta in their centre, contributing with 50% and 71% of the patients included in "AIMS", respectively. A potential selection bias can be excluded for these 15 centres and with a high probability also regarding the total population of "AIMS" since they contributed more than 70% of all patients to the survey. The dialysis patients included in the "AIMS" survey were found to be representative for the dialysis population in Switzerland, also due to the fact that a large number of dialysis patients were included, representing more than 10% (n=368 patients whereof 340 eligible) of the total dialysis population in Switzerland.

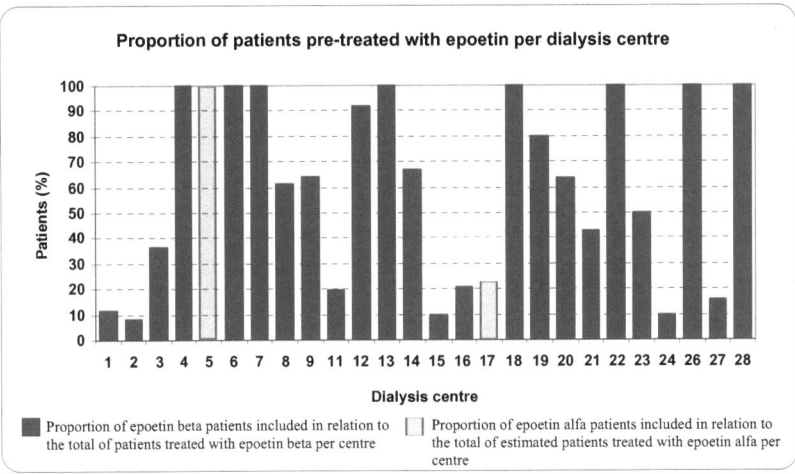

Figure 3-1: Proportion of the survey population pre-treated with epoetin beta in relation to all epoetin beta patients per dialysis centre

Further evidence for representativity was also given by the fact that the prevalence of diagnosis and co-morbidities of patients included in "AIMS" corresponded to those of the European [28] (see Figure 3-2) and US registry database [30]. Nevertheless, the included dialysis patients in "AIMS" were not a random sample; they were representative for the dialysis population in Switzerland.

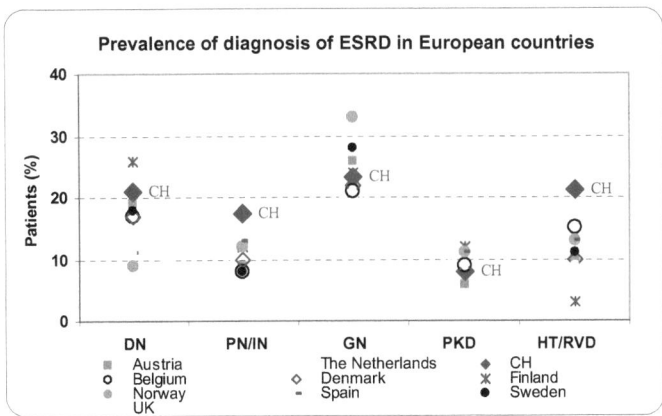

Abbreviations: DN= diabetic nephropathy; PN/IN= pyelonephritis, interstitial nephritis; GN= glomerulonephritis; PKD=polycystic kidney disease; HT/RVD= Hypertension/ renal vascular disease.

Figure 3-2: Prevalence of diagnosis of ESRD in ERA-EDTA countries compared to "AIMS"

3.8 Baseline characteristics

3.8.1 Participating dialysis centres and treatment population

Six months data were analysed of the "AIMS" survey and are presented in this work. 28 of a total of 70 contacted dialysis centres participated in the "AIMS" survey. Eligible data were available from 26 dialysis centres. In total, 368 dialysis patients were included, 340 thereof being eligible. Figure 3-3 gives an overview of the participating centres and the number of eligible patients per dialysis centre. Patients from centre number 10 (n=1) and 26 (n=16) were excluded because of missing reports for all six months.

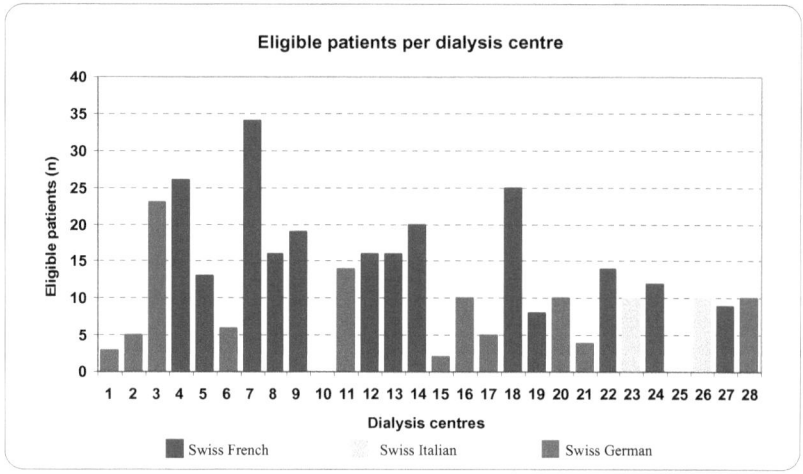

Figure 3-3: Overview of participating dialysis centres and number of eligible patients

The eligible dialysis centres represent a participation rate of 37% of the country's total number of dialysis centres. In total, 14 of 19 dialysis centres of the French speaking part participated in the survey (=participation rate 73.7%) and included 228 eligible patients. In the Swiss German part 12 of totally 47 dialysis centres (=participation rate 25.5%) included 92 eligible patients and of the Italian speaking part 2 of 4 centres (=participation rate 50.0%) included 20 eligible patients. More than 70% of the included patients derived from the Swiss French part because the enrollment proceeded much better in the Swiss French part than previously scheduled.

368 dialyzed patients out of 28 Swiss dialysis centres were included in this survey. Primary variables of 28 patients (haemoglobin and epoetin dosage) were missing for all six months so that the 28 patients were excluded. The remaining treatment population counted 340 dialysis patients and represented 14% of the total dialysis population (=2,483 dialysis patients according to the source of SVK, as of 31.12.2002) [22]. All the analyses were performed in the 340 eligible patients. Table 3-3 provides an overview of the reasons for survey exclusion and the remaining treatment population.

Reasons for survey exclusion	Dialysis centre (number of patients)	Total number of excluded patients	Remaining treatment population
Missing reports of all six months	25 (16)	16	352
Patient with missing primary parameters for all six months	2 (1) 3 (2) 4 (1) 7 (2) 10 (1) 12(1) 14 (1) 16 (1) 19 (1) 27 (1)	12	340
Total		28	340

Table 3-3: Treatment population

Complete data for all six months were available for 299 patients and were not completed for all six months for 41 patients. 21 patients interrupted the survey due to the following reasons: transplantation (n=7 patients), death (n=13 patients), transfer to another dialysis centre (n=7 patients), survey medication interruption/change (n=4 patients) and other/ unknown reasons (n=10 patients). Missing values of haemoglobin, body weight, dosage of epoetin beta, administration frequency, and iron status of those patients were replaced by using the last observation carried forward method (LOCF).

Reasons for interruption	Transplantation (n)	Death (n)	Other reason (n)	Total (n, %)	Cumulative (n, %)
Month 1	0	0	0	0	0
Month 2	2	3	2	7 (2.1)	7 (17.1)
Month 3	1	6	2	9 (2.6)	16 (39.0)
Month 4	3	2	13	18 (5.2)	34 (82.9)
Month 5	1	1	3	5 (1.5)	39 (95.1)
Month 6	0	1	1	2 (0.6)	41 (100)
Total	7	13	21	41 (12.1)	41 (100)

End of each month

Table 3-4: Overview of survey interruption

3.8.2 Patient characteristics

Demographics and baseline parameters of dialysis patients in "AIMS"

All analyses were performed in the eligible treatment population consisting of 340 dialysis patients. 95% of the patients were under haemodialysis and 5% under peritoneal dialysis. Mean age of the studied population was 63.5 ± 14.6 years, ranging from 18-91 years. 58% of the population were male, 42% were female. Dialysis patients represent an elderly patient population, as it is depicted in Figure 3-4 [1, 126]. More than 70% of the survey population were over 60 years old. At survey inclusion, 94.7% of the eligible patients (n=322) received epoetin before study entry and 5.3% of the patients (n=18) were epoetin-naïve with epoetin treatment initiation at patient inclusion.

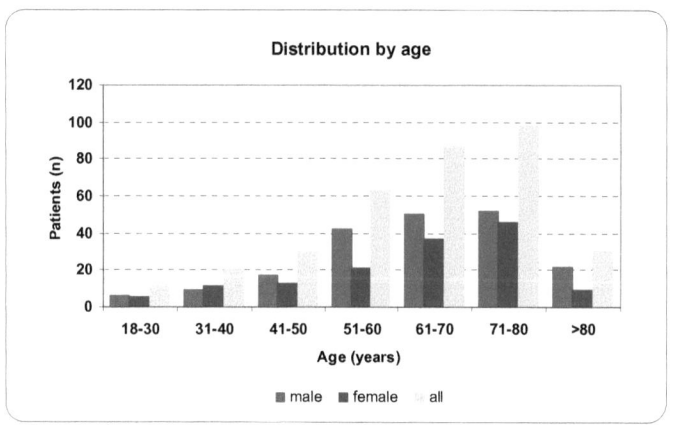

Figure 3-4: Distribution of the eligible population by age

At baseline, mean haemoglobin level was 11.8 ± 1.4 g/dl with a median value of 11.9 g/dl. The 95% confidence interval was between 11.6 and 11.9 g/dl. Haemoglobin levels ranged from 6.6 at lowest to 16.7 g/dl at highest.

Variables at baseline	n	%	Mean ± SD	Median	Confidence interval
Age (years) Range	340		63.5 ± 14.7 18-91	67.0	
Female Male	142 198	41.8 58.2			
Haemodialysis Peritoneal dialysis	324 16	95.3 4.7			
Body weight (kg) Range	340		69.5 ± 15.3 40-129	67.3	67.9-71.2
Systolic blood pressure (mmHg) Diastolic blood pressure (mmHg)	120		161± 23 86 ± 16	160 85	157-166 83-89
Haemoglobin (g/dl) Range	340		11.8 ± 1.4 6.8-15.5	11.9	11.6-11.9
Serum ferritin (µg/l)	340		412 ± 297	402	380-443
Transferrin saturation (%)	245		31 ± 15	27	29-33
Creatinine (µmol/l)	307		692 ± 195	683	670 -714

Table 3-5: Demographics of the treatment population in "AIMS"

Baseline serum ferritin was 411 ± 297 µg/l (95% CI: 380 µg/l to 443 µg/l) and baseline transferrin saturation of available values was 31 ± 15% (n=171). Mean blood pressure at baseline was 161 ± 23 and 86 ± 16 mmHg. A summary of the baseline data is shown in Table 3-5.

Diagnosis of dialysis patients in "AIMS"

The diagnosis of end-stage renal disease of patients included in "AIMS" were diabetic nephropathy in 20.9% (n=71 patients), glomerulonephritis in 23.2% (n=79 patients), interstitial nephritis and pyelonephritis in 17.1% (n=58 patients), hypertension and vascular causes in 21.2% (n=72 patients), polycystic kidney disease in 7.9% (n=27 patients) and tumours in 2.6% (n=9 patients).

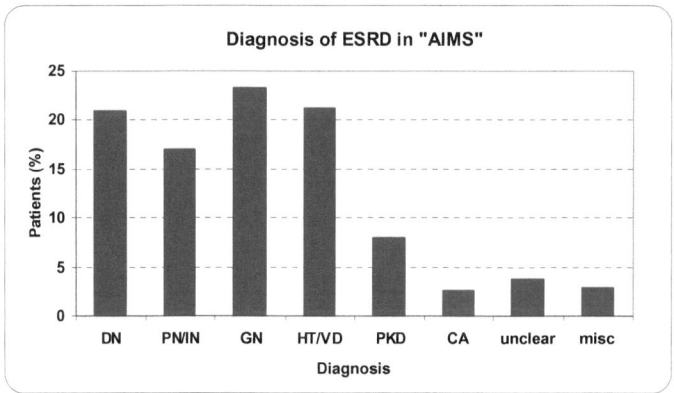

Abbreviations: DN=diabetic nephropathy; PN/IN=pyelonephritis, interstitial nephritis; GN=glomerulonephritis; HT/VD=Hypertension, vascular disease; PKD=polycystic kidney disease; CA=Carcinoma; misc=miscellaneous causes. Multiple entries possible, therefore not cumulative.

Figure 3-5: Diagnosis of end-stage renal disease in "AIMS"

Unclear aetiology was reported in 13 patients (5.4%), and in 9 patients no diagnosis (2.6%) was registered. Figure 3-5 illustrates the diagnosis for chronic kidney disease of patients included in "AIMS". A more detailed overview is provided in Table 3-6.

Co-morbidities of dialysis patients in "AIMS"

Dialysis patients are generally multi-morbid patients. In more than half of the patients, two or more co-morbidities were reported. In 151 patients (=44.4%) two concomitant diseases and in 55 patients (=16.2%) three concomitant diseases were reported. In 12.9% of the patients (n=44 patients) no concomitant disease was reported. Most of the prevalent co-morbidities in this survey were cardiac-related. Hypertension occurred in 60.6% of the patients (n=206 patients), coronary artery disease in 25.5% (n=87 patients) and heart failure in 16.5% (n=56 patients). Diabetes as concomitant disease was reported in 23.2% (n= 79 patients) and miscellaneous causes in 25.9% (n=88 patients). In total, 27.4% (n=93 patients) of the patients were diabetics (either reported as diagnosis or co-morbidity).

Figure 3-6 illustrates the prevalence of concomitant diseases. A more detailed overview is given in Table 3-7.

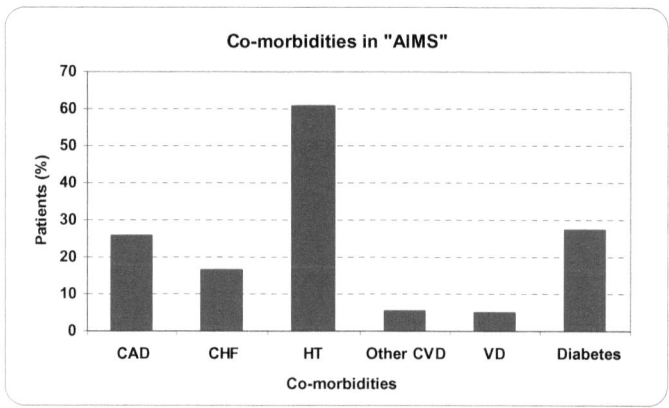

Abbreviations: CAD=coronary artery disease; CHF=congestive heart failure; HT=hypertension; other CVD=other cardiovascular diseases; VD=vascular diseases

Figure 3-6: Co-morbidities in "AIMS" at baseline

As Table 3-7 illustrates, hypertension was the most frequent concomitant disease. Diabetes was reported in ¼ of all elderly dialysis patients (> 50 years) and the risk was 3.45 fold elevated compared to the younger patient group (≤ 50 years). A positive linear correlation was observed between coronary artery disease and age (r^2=0.889) and between heart failure and age (r^2=0.873). Coronary artery disease and heart failure occurred more frequently in patients older than 50 years. The prevalence of hypertension was equally distributed over all age groups.

Diagnosis	Patients		Number of diagnoses	Mean age ± SD (Range)	Sex	
	n	%			Male	female
Diabetic nephropathy	71	20.9	71	64.2 ± 11.7 (21-85)	43	28
Glomerulonephritis	79	23.2	84	59.4 ± 14.7 (18-91)	47	32
Glomerulonephritis			68			
IgA nephropathy, Berger			4			
Hyalinose			2			
Lupus erythematosus			1			
Wegener			1			
Haemolytic uremic syndrome			1			
Vasculitis			4			
Nephrotic syndrome			3			
Pyelonephritis / interstitial nephritis (PN/IN)	58	17.1	61	62.9 ± 13.5 (28-86)	24	34
Chronic PN/IN			48			
Reflux nephritis			7			
Analgesic abuse			5			
Nephrolithiasis			1			
Hypertension / vascular causes	72	21.2	79	69.0 ± 12.4 (34-88)	49	23
Glomerulosclerosis, nephro-angiosclerosis, vascular			58			
hypertension			21			
Polycystic kidney disease (PKD)	27	7.9	27	59.4 ±15.6	11	16
Neoplasm / tumours	9	2.6	9	67.3 ± 11.2 (46-83)	5	4
Amyloidosis			3			
Renal neoplasm			1			
Multiple myeloma			1			
Adenocarcinoma			1			
Other carcinoma			3			
Unclear /multifactorial	13	3.8	13	62.7 ± 16.8 (34-82)	8	5
Miscellaneous causes	10	2.9	10	55.6 ± 23.2 (31-81)	5	5
Thalassemia			1			
HIV			1			
Tx			2			
Hydronephrosis / hypoplasia / atrophia			3			
Other renal disorders (Bricker, polynephritis)			3			
Missing	9	2.6	-	62.2 ± 19.2 (22-80)	8	1

Multiple entries possible, therefore not cumulative.

Table 3-6: Reported diagnosis of end-stage renal disease in "AIMS"

Concomitant diseases	Patients		Mean age ± SD	Range	Sex	
	n	%			male	female
Coronary artery disease	87	25.5	67.0 ± 11.8	22-88	58	29
Congestive heart failure	56	16.5	67.8 ± 11.0	22-84	37	19
Hypertension	206	60.6	63.9 ± 15.0	18-91	112	94
Other cardiac diseases[1]	18	5.3	65.8 ±14.1	30-87	9	9
Diabetes[2]	93	27.4	65.3 ± 11.1	34-85	59	34
Vascular diseases[3]	17	5.0	67.7 ± 8.7	53-90	8	9
Metabolic disorders[4]	7	2.0	61.0 ± 15.3	34-78	2	5
Hyperparathyroidism	6	1.8	56.2 ± 20.9	21-83	3	3
Nephrectomia / CsA Nephropathy / -sclerosis	3	0.9	58.7 ± 13.5	45-72	2	1
Pulmonary diseases (COPD)	6	1.8	61.8 ± 16.8	30-74	1	5
Hepatological disorders[5]	7	2.0	52.4 ± 10.5	37-67	4	3
Cancer (CA)[6]	7	2.0	69.7 ± 13.6	46-85	6	1
Bone diseases[7]	4	1.2	70.5 ± 12.7	56-87	1	3
Other diseases[8]	7	2.0	59.6 ± 20.5	33-87	3	4

[1] Aneurism (2); Mitral insufficiency (2); Paroxysmal tachycardia (1); Pericarditis (1); Valvulopathy (2); Replacement of aortic valvae (1) Ischemic cardiomyopathy (9)
[2] Diabetes (overall): thereof reported as primary diagnosis (n= 71 patients)
[3] Arteriosclerosis, arteriopathy, polyarteriovascular disease (12); Cerebrovascular disorder (3); Haemorrhagia (2);
[4] Adipositas (3); Hypercholesterolemia (1); Thyroiditis (1); Gout (2)
[5] Liver transplantation (1); Liver cirrhosis (4); Pancreatitis (2)
[6] Prostate CA (2); Amyloidosis (1); ORL CA (1); Stomach CA (1); others (2)
[7] Osteoporosis (1); Polyarthitis (3)
[8] Psoriasis (1); Thalassemia (1); Diverticulitis (1); Epilepsy (1); Paraplegia (1); Morbus Crohn (1); Dementia (1)
(in brackets: number of patients)
Multiple entries possible, therefore not cumulative.

Table 3-7: Reported concomitant diseases in "AIMS"

3.9 Summary

The eligible dialysis centres represent 37% of the country's total number of dialysis centres. Dialysis centres of all three geographical parts of Switzerland with a higher proportion of dialysis centres from the Swiss French part participated at the survey. The dialysis patients included in "AIMS" were representative for the total Swiss dialysis population.

368 patients were included in this survey, with 340 of them being eligible. Dialysis patients were mainly at middle or advanced age. Main diagnoses of ESRD in "AIMS" were glomerulonephritis (23%), diabetic nephropathy (21%) and vascular diseases (21%). Dialysis patients are generally multi-morbid patients. End-stage renal disease was accompanied by two or more co-morbidities in more than half of the patients included in "AIMS". About 80-90% of patients with renal insufficiency suffered from anaemia at dialysis start. Baseline haemoglobin was 11.8 g/dl in "AIMS" and corresponded for the majority of the patients to the recommendations of the EBPG.

4. Anaemia Management in dialysis patients in Switzerland "AIMS": Assessment of the quality of anaemia control achieved with epoetin beta in dialysis patients in Switzerland

N. Lötscher[1,2], D. Teta[3], D. Kiss[4], P.-Y. Martin[5], L. Gabutti[6], M. Burnier[3*]

1   Roche (Pharma) Switzerland Ltd, P.O. Box, CH-4153 Reinach, Switzerland
2   Swiss Tropical Institute, Department of Public Health and Epidemiology, P.O. Box, CH-4002 Basel, Switzerland
3   CHUV, Department of Internal Medicine, Nephrology, P.O. Box, CH-1011 Lausanne, Switzerland
4   Kantonsspital Liestal, Department of Nephrology, P.O. Box, CH-4410 Liestal, Switzerland
5   HCUG, Department of Internal Medicine, Nephrology, P.O. Box, CH-1211 Geneva, Switzerland
6   Ospedale regionale La Carità, Department of Nephrology, P.O. Box, CH-6601 Locarno, Switzerland

*Corresponding author:

Tel.:   +41 21 314 11 54
E-mail: michel.burnier@hospvd.ch

Working paper to be submitted

4.1 Abstract

Aim: The purpose of this survey was to evaluate the quality of the anaemia control obtained with epoetin beta in Switzerland. It was the first large scale survey in Switzerland to assess clinical practice of anaemia treatment in dialysis patients after the edition of the EBPG.
Method: 368 dialyzed patients of 28 dialysis centres in Switzerland were included in this non-randomized practice-based, open-intervention survey, 340 thereof were eligible [58% male, 42% female, medium age 64 years, mostly (n=322) pre-treated with epoetin]. Anaemia treatment with epoetin beta in clinical practice was observed for 12 months. Efficacy, frequency and route of administration of epoetin beta as well as serum ferritin were documented monthly. Hyporesponse to epoetin beta treatment was assessed according to achieved serum ferritin levels.
Results: Six months data are presented in this article. The analysis was performed in 340 patients. Mean haemoglobin levels at baseline and month 1, 2, 3, 4, 5 and 6 were 11.8 ± 1.4, 11.7 ± 1.3, 11.7 ± 1.4, 11.8 ± 1.4, 11.9 ± 1.3, 11.8 ±1.4 and 11.8 ±1.4 g/dl, respectively. Lowest haemoglobin value was 6.6 g/dl and highest 16.7 g/dl. At baseline and month 6, 74% and 76% of the treatment population achieved haemoglobin levels ≥11 g/dl; 46% and 49%, respectively, achieved haemoglobin levels ≥12 g/dl. Mean weekly epoetin beta dose at baseline and at month 6 was 143 ± 108 (median: 116) and 155 ± 126 (median: 119) IU/kg/week, respectively. At baseline and at month 6, mean weekly epoetin dose was less than 200 IU/kg/week in 78% and 77% of the patients, respectively. At baseline, epoetin beta was administered in 71% of the patients 1x weekly, in 21% 2x weekly and in 7% 3x weekly. 71% of the patients received epoetin beta subcutaneously at baseline, with no major change during the survey. 60.9% of the patients received epoetin beta as a 1x weekly dosing regimen for all six months. Subcutaneous administration of epoetin beta resulted in significantly higher haemoglobin levels for month 1-6 compared to intravenous administration, with no differences in epoetin doses. Baseline serum ferritin was 412 ± 297 µg/l and remained stable throughout the study. An inverse relationship was found between epoetin dose and haemoglobin level. Mean haemoglobin levels were significantly lower in patients with mean weekly epoetin doses ≥200 and ≥300 IU/kg/week than in patients with mean weekly epoetin doses <200 and <300 IU/kg/week, respectively. At baseline, serum ferritin deficiency was found to be responsible for non-response to epoetin treatment.
Conclusions: Anaemia management was well controlled and a high quality of anaemia control was achieved in dialysis patients in Switzerland. Epoetin beta was predominantly administered as a 1x weekly dosing regimen. It can be administered by different routes of administration and dosing frequencies, allowing individualized anaemia therapy. Anaemia treatment improved over the last five years towards higher haemoglobin level.

Key words: Anaemia, anaemia management, epoetin, epoetin beta, dosing frequency, end-stage renal disease, dialysis

4.2 Introduction

Over 90% of chronic kidney disease (CKD) patients on dialysis develop anaemia. Anaemia progressively worsens as renal function declines and correlates inversely with residual renal function. Anaemia is prevalent in a considerable number of patients long before they are on dialysis. Anaemia has been found to be an independent risk factor for cardiovascular morbidity and mortality [3, 31]. The introduction of recombinant erythropoietin (rHuEPO) over more than 15 years ago has revolutionized anaemia treatment in dialysis patients and made it the first effective treatment for anaemia in chronic renal insufficiency [127]. Treatment of CKD with epoetin leads to an increase in haemoglobin level and improves anaemia-related symptoms. The process of defining optimal dosage regimens, different routes of administration and optimal iron treatment lasted nearly ten years and is still ongoing. There are still unanswered questions, such as the optimal target haemoglobin, current anaemia treatment in clinical practice, identification of clinical predictors and the long-term effect of anaemia correction.

Over the last decade, new findings have successively influenced anaemia treatment of chronic kidney disease. Epoetin was first administered 3-7 times a week intravenously. Since several studies have demonstrated a greater efficacy of the subcutaneous administration compared to intravenous administration, allowing target haemoglobin levels to be reached with epoetin doses lowered by 20-30%, epoetin became predominantly used subcutaneously [74, 128, 129]. Subcutaneous administration of epoetin resulted in a longer half-life time and a delayed absorption, which allowed to increase the dosing intervals with adequate therapeutic levels of epoetin [77-79, 90]. Epoetin treatment was found to be effective and well tolerated with few side effects. In 2002, serious concerns about safety of epoetin have been raised leading to the contraindication of subcutaneous administration of epoetin alfa [86]. This might have had major implications on physicians' clinical practice of anaemia treatment in chronic kidney disease patients, since anaemia treatment of chronic kidney disease progressively changes over time due to new findings or clinical experiences and needs, beside available guidelines, periodic re-evaluation.

In the US, anaemia treatment, diagnosis and concomitant disease are annually registered and published in the USRDS annual report [1]. In Europe, selected countries provide data to the ERA-EDTA registry. Some countries, such as England or Germany, run country-based registries [126]. However, in Switzerland, registry database for chronic kidney disease has not yet been established and, in contrast to other countries, anaemia management for this population has never been regularly assessed [12, 130]. Even though anaemia management in dialysis patients was assessed in a large survey (ESAM) throughout Europe in 1998 [119], results had hardly been analysed per country and may have changed over the last five years. The present survey was the first survey in Switzerland assessing current anaemia management and the quality of control of anaemia management at a larger scale after the publication of the EBPG in 1998.

The primary objective of this survey was to assess the quality of the anaemia control with epoetin beta and current anaemia treatment in dialysis patients in Switzerland. The effectiveness of epoetin beta, the predominant application frequency and route of administration was assessed in dialysis patients. Hyporesponsiveness and iron status were investigated as secondary parameters.

4.3 Subjects and methods

Patients and data collection

The survey was a prospective, open-intervention, non-randomized survey with the objective to assess anaemia management in dialysis patients in Switzerland. The survey was conducted under the acronym "AIMS" and stands for *AnaemIa Management* in dialysis patients in *S*witzerland. 368 dialysis patients of 28 Swiss dialysis centres were included in this survey, 340 patients thereof were eligible. Patient recruitment lasted from June 2002 until December 2003, with an observation period of 12 months.

Inclusion criteria were dialysis patients (≥ 18 years old) either on haemodialysis or peritoneal dialysis with presence of renal anaemia being under epoetin therapy or epoetin-naïve patients. Exclusion criteria were defined according to the contraindication of the product information of epoetin and included patients with unstable angina pectoris, untreated hypertension, haemoglobinopathy, haemolysis, epilepsy, pregnancy or lactation. Patients had to be iron-replete (≥ 200 µg/l) and without any deficiency of vitamin B_{12} or folic acid.

At patient registration, baseline parameters and patient characteristics were registered. Anaemia management was documented over a time period of 12 months. Epoetin beta dosage and haemoglobin were registered at baseline and from month 1 to 12. No interference or change of treatment strategies was requested, as the aim of the survey was to assess current anaemia management with epoetin beta in Switzerland. For this kind of survey no approval of the ethical committees was requested. Patient did not need to sign an informed consent sheet.

The survey was presented to 70 dialysis centres whereof 28 centres participated. Patients from 26 centres were eligible. At patient registration (baseline), aetiology of chronic renal failure, concomitant diseases (coronary artery disease, diabetes, heart failure, hypertension and others), dialysis modality, dry weight and laboratory parameter, such as haemoglobin, serum ferritin, transferrin saturation and serum creatinine were registered. Laboratory parameters were documented if performed in the course of the clinical routine. Epoetin beta treatment (weekly dose, frequency and route of administration) and haemoglobin concentration were monthly assessed. Serum ferritin and transferrin saturation were documented, if performed. The schedule of assessments is depicted in Table 4-1.

Schedule of assessments	Baseline	Monthly reports (M1–M12)	Final report (M12 or at survey interruption)
Medical history	x		
Weight	x	x	
Blood pressure	x		
Epoetin treatment	x		
Concomitant anaemia treatment	x	x	
Epoetin beta dose/frequency	x	x	
Route of administration	x	x	
Adverse events		x	
Laboratory data			
– haemoglobin	x	x	
– transferrin saturation	x	x	
– ferritin*	x	x	
– creatinine*	x	x	
Assessment of efficacy and practicability	x	x	x

*where available

Table 4-1: Schedule of assessments

The received filled-in data report forms were examined regarding to completeness of mandatory data and validated prior to data entry. Mandatory data for patients were patient's dry weight, haemoglobin, epoetin dose, route of administration and administration frequency of epoetin beta. Mean weekly epoetin beta dose per kilogram body weight (IU/kg/week) was calculated using the following formula:

$$\text{Epoetin/kg/week} = \frac{\text{Epoetin beta [IU]} * \text{administration frequency per week}}{\text{Body weight [kg]}}$$

All patients who received at least one dose of epoetin beta were included in the analysis. Centres were contacted if mandatory values were missing. Missing values (haemoglobin, body weight, epoetin beta dose, administration frequency, route of administration) of patients, who received at least one survey medication, were replaced by using the last observation carried forward method (LOCF). Non-mandatory data, such as serum ferritin, transferrin saturation and serum creatinine, were requested to fill in, if performed. Some of the non-mandatory data were not available for all 340 patients (=shown in analysis as unknown or missing). All data deriving from the report forms were entered by using excel database (Excel 2002).

Statistics

Simple statistical analyses were performed in Excel 2002 or Epi-Info®, version 3.2. Complex statistics were performed using the SAS statistical program version 8.2 (SAS, Institute, Cary, NC, USA). Standard descriptive statistics (mean, standard deviation, confidence interval) were calculated for all variables including haemoglobin, epoetin dose, administration frequency and route of administration. Categorical variables were presented in absolute number and percentage. Categorical variables were compared with the χ^2-test and continuous variables with the Student's t-test or Wilcoxon two-sample test, where appropriate. All statistical tests were two-sided and the significance was proofed on a 0.05 p-level.

4.4 Results

28 participating dialysis centres (=40%) included 368 patients, 340 patients thereof from 26 centres were eligible, representing 37 % of the total dialysis centres in Switzerland. 28 patients were excluded from the survey due to missing efficacy parameters for the total observation period. The remaining treatment population counted 340 dialysis patients and represented 14 % of the total dialysis population. The analysis was performed on these 340 eligible dialysis patients. Table 3-3, page 47 provides an overview of patient exclusion. Six months data are presented in this article.

4.4.1 Patient characteristics

324 patients (95%) were on haemodialysis and 16 patients (5%) on peritoneal dialysis. 142 of the eligible patients (42%) were female and 198 patients (58%) were male. US registry data also revealed a similar picture where more males (54.5%) than females (45.5%) required renal replacement therapy as well [1, 30]. Mean age was 63.5 ± 14.7 years (median age: 67 years) with more than 70% of the patients older than 60 years. Mean age for males and females was 63.8 ± 14.3 years and 63.1 ± 27.7 years, respectively (p=0.62, Students't-test). In the age group of 51-60 years significantly more dialysis patients were male (21.2%) than female (p=0.08, χ^2-test). In the age group of 71-80 years more dialysis patients were female (32.4%) than male (26.3%) without significant difference (p=1.52; χ^2-test). Mean body weight was 69.5 ± 15.3 kg and ranged from 40 to 129 kg (95% confidence interval: 67.9-71.2 kg). Mean systolic and diastolic blood pressure was 161 ± 23 mmHg and 86 ± 16 mmHg. Systolic blood pressure (≥ 140 mmHg) was elevated in 80% of the patients (n=120). Baseline variables are shown in Table 4-2. Most common diagnoses of end-stage renal disease were glomerulonephritis (23.2%), diabetic nephropathy (20.9%), hypertension and vascular diseases (21.2%), polycystic kidney disease (7.9%) and tumours (2.6%). More details are provided in Table 3-6, page 51. In more than half of the patients two or more co-morbidities were reported. Most frequently registered co-morbidities were cardiac-related. Coronary artery disease was

registered in 25.5%, congestive heart failure in 16.5%, and hypertension in 60.6% of the patients. Diabetes was reported in 93 patients. A detailed overview is given in Table 3-7, page 52.

Variable at baseline	n	%	Mean ± SD	Median	Confidence interval
Age (years) Range	340		63.5 ± 14.7 18-91	67.0	
Female Male	142 198	41.8 58.2			
Haemodialysis Peritoneal dialysis	324 16	95.3 4.7			
Body weight (kg) Range	340		69.5 ± 15.3 40-129	67.3	67.9-71.2
Haemoglobin (g/dl) Range	340		11.8 ± 1.4 6.8-15.5	11.9	11.6-11.9
Serum ferritin (µg/l)	340		412 ± 297	402	380-443
Transferrin saturation (%)	245		31 ± 15	27	29-33

Table 4-2: Baseline parameters

4.4.2 Anaemia treatment with epoetin beta

Haemoglobin

At baseline and month 6, mean haemoglobin was 11.8 ± 1.4 g/dl (95% CI: 11.6-11.9 g/dl) and 11.8 ± 1.4 g/dl (95% CI: 11.7-12.0 g/dl), respectively. No significant shift in haemoglobin distribution was observed between baseline and month 6, as illustrated in Figure 4-1 (p= 0.492, Student's t-test).

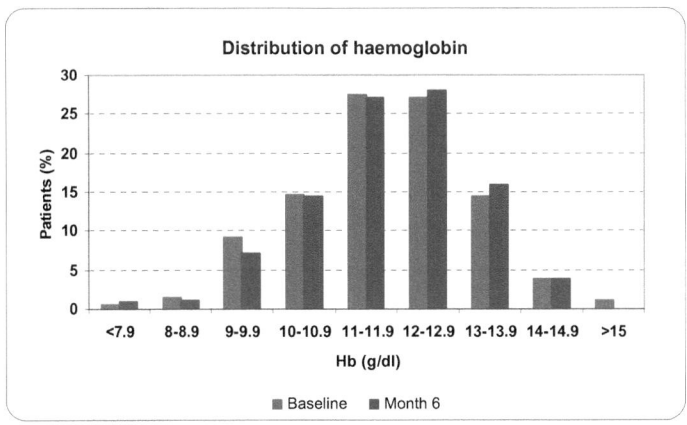

Figure 4-1: Distribution of haemoglobin at baseline and month 6

Mean haemoglobin at baseline and month 1, 2, 3, 4, 5 and 6 were 11.8 ± 1.4 g/dl (95% CI: 11.6-11.9), 11.7 ± 1.4 g/dl (95% CI: 11.6-11.9), 11.7 ± 1.4 g/dl (95% CI: 11.6-11.9), 11.8 ± 1.4 g/dl (95% CI: 11.6-11.9), 11.9 ± 1.3 g/dl (95% CI: 11.7-12.0), 11.8 ± 1.4 g/dl (95% CI: 11.7-12.0) and 11.8 ± 1.4 g/dl (95% CI: 11.7-12.0), respectively.

Mean haemoglobin level remained stable during the observation period, as illustrated in Figure 4-2. Lowest haemoglobin value was 6.6 g/dl and highest 16.7 g/dl.

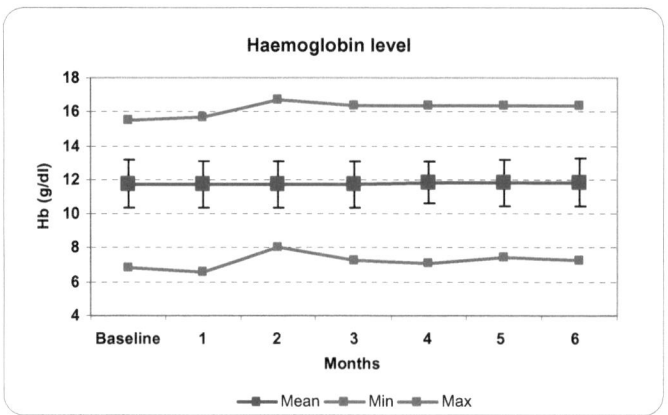

Figure 4-2: Mean haemoglobin levels (± SD) for 6 months

Mean haemoglobin of females and males was plotted versus age and stratified according to age decades (18-30, 31-40, 41-50, 51-60, 61-70, 71-80, 81-90, 91-100). The result is shown in Figure 4-3.

Mean haemoglobin level was on average 0.5 g/dl higher (not significant) in males than in females for the age category of 30-60 years. For patients older than 60 years, mean haemoglobin concentration was at the same level for males and females. Unexpectedly, mean haemoglobin level of young males (<30 years) was lower (10.6 g/dl) than of females (11.3 g/dl) in the age category 18-30, which can be explained by the fact that one male patient was epoetin-naïve with a low haemoglobin concentration of 6.6 g/dl at baseline. There was also a trend towards lower haemoglobin level with increasing age.

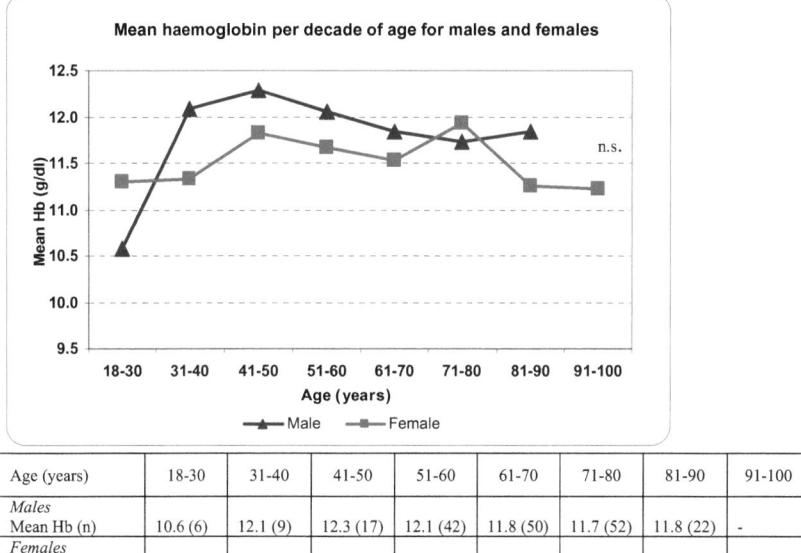

Age (years)	18-30	31-40	41-50	51-60	61-70	71-80	81-90	91-100
Males Mean Hb (n)	10.6 (6)	12.1 (9)	12.3 (17)	12.1 (42)	11.8 (50)	11.7 (52)	11.8 (22)	-
Females Mean Hb (n)	11.3 (5)	11.3 (11)	11.8 (13)	11.7 (21)	11.5 (37)	11.9 (46)	11.3 (8)	11.2 (1)

n.s.=not significant

Figure 4-3: Mean haemoglobin per decade of age for males and females

Treatment with epoetin beta

94.7 % (n=322) of the patients included in "AIMS" were pre-treated with epoetin and 5.3% (n=18) were epoetin-naïve patients. 77.6% (n=250 patients) of the patients pre-treated with epoetin received epoetin beta at survey inclusion, 19.3% epoetin alfa (n= 62 patients) and 1.9% epoetin alfa and/or epoetin beta (n= 6 patients). Of 4 patients, epoetin pre-treatment was unknown.

At baseline and after month 1 on to month 6, mean weekly epoetin beta dose was 143 ± 108 IU/kg/week (95% CI: 132-155 IU/kg/week), 143 ± 106 IU/kg/week (95% CI: 132-154 IU/kg/week), 151 ± 117 IU/kg/week (95% CI: 139-164 IU/kg/week), 151 ± 120 IU/kg/week (95% CI: 139-164 IU/kg/week), 152 ± 127 IU/kg/week (95% CI: 139–166 IU/kg/week), 152 ± 124 IU/kg/week (95% CI: 139-166 IU/kg/week) and 155 ± 126 IU/kg/week (95% CI: 142-169 IU/kg/week), respectively.

Mean and median weekly epoetin beta dosages during the six months observation period are illustrated in Figure 4-4. The median weekly epoetin beta dose was lower than the mean weekly epoetin beta and was at baseline and at month 1 to 6 116 IU/kg/week, 114 IU/kg/week, 121 IU/kg/week, 119 IU/kg/week, 121 IU/kg/week, 120 IU/kg/week and 119 IU/kg/week, respectively.

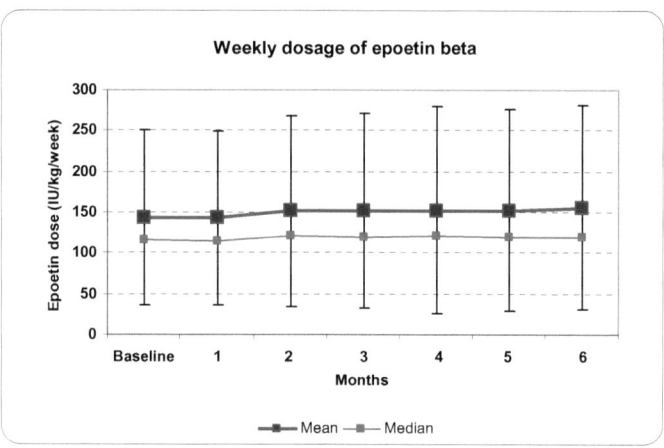

Figure 4-4: Mean (± SD) and median weekly dosage of epoetin beta for 6 months

At baseline and after 6 months, 44.7 % and 43.9% of the patients received mean weekly epoetin beta doses (IU/kg/week) of less than 100 IU/kg per week, respectively, and 78.5% and 77.3% of the patients received less than 200 IU/kg, respectively.

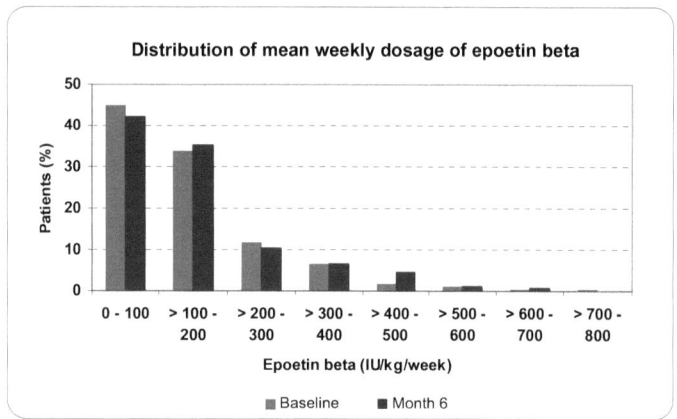

Figure 4-5: Distribution of mean weekly dosage of epoetin beta per kg (IU/kg)

In 66.2 % of the patients, less than 200 IU/kg/week epoetin beta dose was necessary to achieve target haemoglobin of ≥11 g/dl. At baseline, 45% of all patients received between 1,000 and 6,000 IU epoetin beta per week and 74% less than 10,000 IU epoetin beta per week.

Administration frequency of epoetin beta

At baseline, 71% of the patients received epoetin beta 1x weekly, 21% twice weekly and 7% three times weekly. One patient received epoetin beta every other week. After month 6, 73% of the patients received epoetin beta 1x weekly, 20% twice weekly and 7% three times weekly.

Figure 4-6 provides an overview of the administration frequencies of epoetin beta at baseline and after month 6.

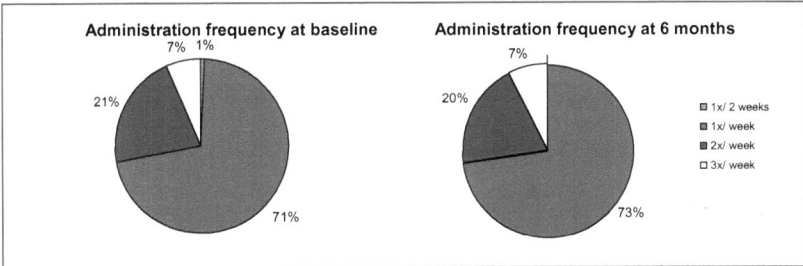

Figure 4-6: Administration frequency of epoetin beta at baseline and after month 6

The dosing frequency of epoetin beta was switched from a 1x weekly to a 2-3x weekly administration frequency in about 10% of the patients. 60.9% of the patients received epoetin beta as a 1x weekly dosing regimen for all 6 months (n=207 patients).

Route of administration of epoetin beta

At baseline, 70.9% of the patients received epoetin beta subcutaneously and 29.1% intravenously. At month 6, 69.4% of the patients received epoetin beta subcutaneously and 30.6% intravenously. No significant shift in the selection of the route of administration occurred during the observation period. The route of administration stratified according to the dosing frequency is illustrated in Table 4-3. At baseline and at month 6, 73.4% of the 1x weekly patient group received epoetin beta subcutaneously. In the 2-3x weekly group, 66.9% and 63.2% of the patients received epoetin beta subcutaneously at baseline and at month 6, respectively. A small but not significant shift towards the intravenous administration was observed for patients receiving epoetin beta 2-3x weekly.

	Baseline n		Month 6 n		Baseline %		Month 6 %	
	s.c.	i.v.	s.c.	i.v.	s.c.	i.v.	s.c.	i.v.
Overall	241	99	236	104	70.9	29.1	69.4	30.6
1x weekly (n=207)	152	55	152	55	73.4	26.6	73.4	26.6
2-3x weekly (n=133)	89	44	84	49	66.9	33.1	63.2	36.8

Table 4-3: Route of administration listed by dosing frequency

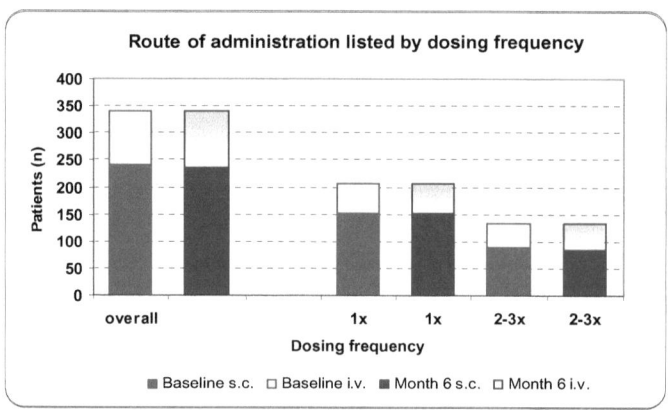

Figure 4-7: Route of administration listed by dosing frequency

Efficacy of subcutaneous and intravenous administration of epoetin beta

Two third of the patients received epoetin beta subcutaneously and one third intravenously. At baseline, 241 patients received epoetin beta subcutaneously and 99 patients intravenously. This proportion slightly changed over the six months in favour of the intravenous route of administration. Efficacy parameters of epoetin beta (mean weekly epoetin beta dose and haemoglobin) and the proportion of patients treated with epoetin beta by route of administration are listed in Table 4-4 .

Route of administration	Number of patients n		Mean weekly epoetin dosage IU/kg/week			Mean haemoglobin g/dl		
	s.c.	i.v.	s.c.	i.v.	p-value	s.c.	i.v.	p value
Baseline	241	99	149	131	0.15	11.8	11.7	0.53
Month 1	241	99	146	135	0.33	11.9	11.3	0.0002
Month 2	235	105	151	151	0.99	11.9	11.3	<0.0001
Month 3	234	106	147	162	0.29	12.0	11.3	<0.0001
Month 4	236	104	151	155	0.71	12.0	11.6	0.007
Month 5	236	104	153	151	0.80	12.0	11.5	0.002
Month 6	236	104	157	153	0.75	12.0	11.5	0.004

Table 4-4: Efficacy of epoetin beta listed by route of administration (s.c. and i.v.)

The efficacy of the subcutaneous versus the intravenous route of administration was analysed in terms of epoetin dose and haemoglobin. At baseline and at month 1 to 6, mean weekly epoetin beta dose of the subcutaneous group was 149 ± 110 IU/kg/week (95% CI: 135-162 IU/kg/week), 146 ± 110 IU/kg/week (95% CI: 132-160 IU/kg/week), 151 ± 118 IU/kg/week (95% CI: 136-166 IU/kg/week), 147 ± 114 IU/kg/week (95% CI: 132-161 IU/kg/week), 151 ± 132 IU/kg/week (95% CI: 134-168 IU/kg/week), 153 ± 133

IU/kg/week (95% CI: 136-170 IU/kg/week) and 157 ± 134 IU/kg/week (95% CI: 139-174 IU/kg/week), respectively. In the intravenous group, mean epoetin dose at baseline and at month 1 to 6 was 131 ± 102 IU/kg/week (95% CI: 110-151 IU/kg/week), 135 ± 95 IU/kg/week (95% CI: 116-154 IU/kg/week), 151 ± 117 IU/kg/week (95% CI: 128-173 IU/kg/week), 162 ± 132 IU/kg/week (95% CI: 137-187 IU/kg/week), 155 ± 114 IU/kg/week (95% CI: 133-177 IU/kg/week), 151 ± 101 IU/kg/week (95% CI: 131-170 IU/kg/week) and 153 ± 105 IU/kg/week (95% CI: 133-173 IU/kg/week), respectively. In contrast to the literature [73, 74], no significant difference was observed at any time of the survey period between the subcutaneous and intravenous group in respect of mean weekly epoetin dose (Figure 4-8).

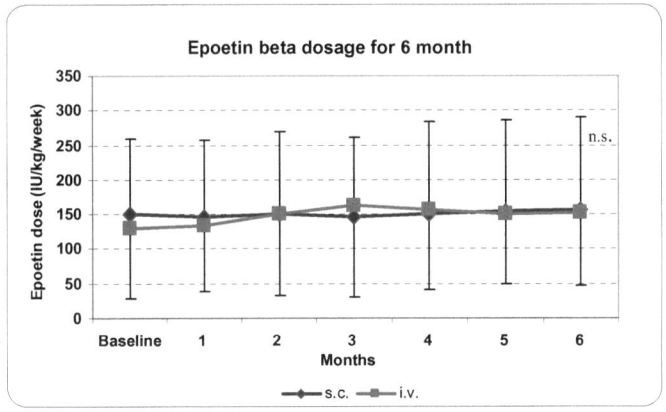

n.s.=not significant

Figure 4-8: Epoetin beta dosage for subcutaneous and intravenous administration for 6 months

In the subcutaneous group, mean weekly haemoglobin concentration at baseline and at month 1 to 6 was 11.8 ± 1.4 g/dl (95% CI: 11.5-12.0 g/dl), 11.9 ±1.4 g/dl (95% CI: 11.7-12.1 g/dl), 11.9 ± 1.3 g/dl (95% CI: 11.7-12.1 g/dl), 12.0 ± 1.3 g/dl (95% CI: 11.8-12.2 g/dl), 12.0 ± 1.2 g/dl (95% CI: 11.8-12.1 g/dl), 12.0 ± 1.3 g/dl (95% CI: 11.8-12.2 g/dl) and 12.0 ± 1.4 g/dl (95% CI: 11.8-12.2 g/dl), respectively.

At baseline and at month 1 to 6, mean weekly haemoglobin concentration in the intravenous group was 11.7 ± 1.4 g/dl (95% CI: 11.3-12.0 g/dl), 11.3 ± 1.2 g/dl (95% CI: 11.0-11.6 g/dl), 11.3 ± 1.4 g/dl (95% CI: 10.9-11.6 g/dl), 11.3 ± 1.4 g/dl (95% CI: 10.9-11.6 g/dl), 11.6 ± 1.3 g/dl (95% CI: 11.2-11.9 g/dl), 11.5 ± 1.4 g/dl (95% CI :11.1-11.8 g/dl) and 11.5 ± 1.4 g/dl (95% CI: 11.2-11.8 g/dl), respectively.

At baseline, no significant difference in haemoglobin concentration was observed between the two groups. Haemoglobin level was significantly lower in the intravenous group compared to the subcutaneous group for month 1 to month 6 (p<0.01; Students' t-test), as illustrated in Figure 4-9. Mean serum ferritin levels were in both groups above 200 µg/l. Mean serum ferritin values ranged in the subcutaneous group between 229-396 µg/l and in the intravenous group between 426-540 µg/l.

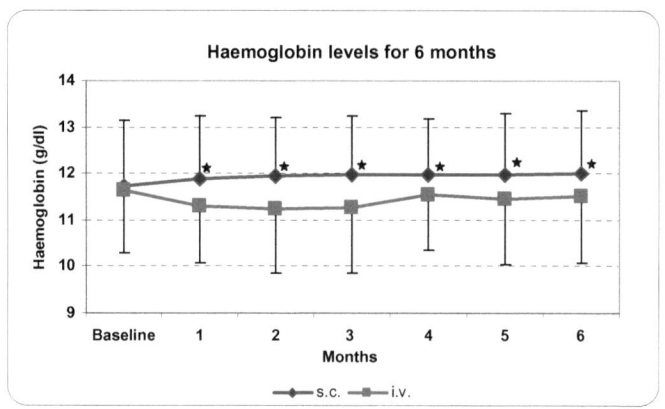

* significant difference

Figure 4-9: Haemoglobin levels (± SD) for s.c. and i.v. administration of epoetin beta

The subcutaneous administration was found to be more efficacious in terms of achieved haemoglobin level than the intravenous administration (observed for month 1 to 6). Comparable epoetin beta doses were administered in both groups.

4.4.3 Iron status

In the "AIMS" survey, mean serum ferritin level was 411 ± 297 µg/l (95% CI: 380-443 µg/l) at baseline and 429 ± 315 µg/l (95% CI: 396-463 µg/l) at month 6, with no significant difference. Mean serum ferritin level remained stable over the six months observation period, as illustrated in Figure 4-10.

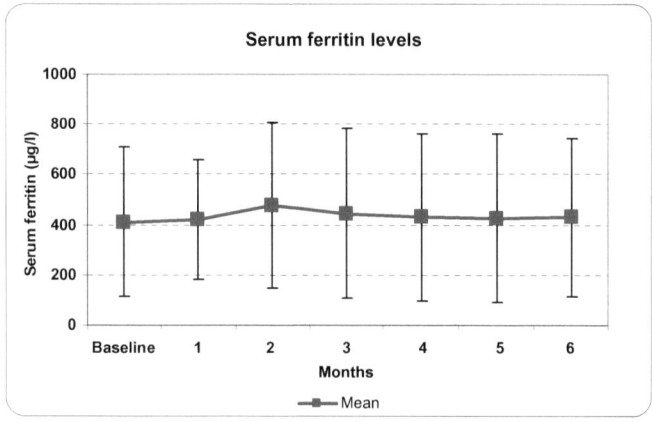

Figure 4-10: Mean serum ferritin levels (±SD)

Mean serum ferritin was 422 ± 240 µg/l at month 1 (95% CI: 396-447 µg/l), 477 ± 328 µg/l at month 2 (95% CI: 442-512 µg/l), 444 ± 337 µg/l at month 3 (95% CI: 408-480 µg/l), 429 ± 333 µg/l at month 4 (95% CI: 394-465 µg/l) and 427 µg/l ± 336 at month 5 (95% CI: 391-463 µg/l).

Mean serum ferritin for females and males were 420 ± 277 µg/l (95% CI: 374-466 µg/l) and 395 ± 251 µg/l (95% CI: 360-430 µg/l), respectively, with no significant difference. Mean serum ferritin was stratified by decades of age (Table 4-5). No significant difference occurred in mean serum ferritin for males and females at each decade of age.

Age (years)	18-30	31-40	41-50	51-60	61-70	71-80	81-90	91-100
Males Mean serum ferritin µg/l (patients)	367 (6)	268 (9)	421 (17)	382 (42)	450 (50)	460 (52)	413 (22)	-
Females Mean serum ferritin µg/l (patients)	413 (5)	433 (11)	481 (13)	417 (21)	437 (37)	497 (46)	381 (8)	375 (1)

Table 4-5: Mean serum ferritin levels listed by age for males and females

Figure 4-11 illustrates the distribution of serum ferritin at baseline and at month 6. The distribution of serum ferritin levels was comparable between baseline and month 6. Serum ferritin level was, in the majority of the patients (92% at baseline; 90% at month 6), above the recommended minimal target level (≥100 µg/l) which is necessary for adequate response to epoetin treatment. Optimal serum ferritin target levels (≥200 µg/l) were achieved in 81% at baseline and in 79% of the patients at month 6. In approximately 10% of the patients (7.6% at baseline; 10% at month 6), mean serum ferritin was lower than the requested minimal serum ferritin level of 100 µg/l. At baseline and at month 6, 57% and 49% of the patients were within the range of 200 and 500 µg/l, respectively.

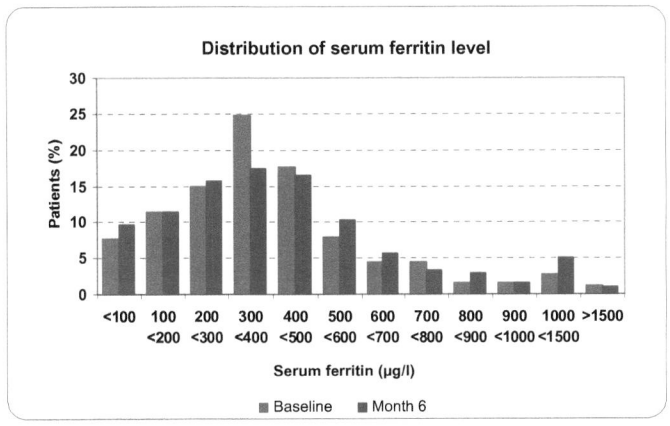

Figure 4-11: Distribution of serum ferritin at baseline and month 6

Serum ferritin	Mean serum ferritin <100 µg/l		Mean serum ferritin ≥100 µg/l		Mean serum ferritin ≥ 200 µg/l	
	Patients n	Patients %	Patients n	Patients %	Patients n	Patients %
Baseline	26	7.6	314	92.3	275	80.9
Month 1	17	5.0	323	95.0	301	88.5
Month 2	24	7.1	316	92.9	289	85.0
Month 3	31	9.1	309	90.9	270	79.4
Month 4	32	9.4	308	90.6	264	77.6
Month 5	33	9.7	307	90.3	265	77.9
Month 6	33	9.7	307	90.3	268	78.8

Table 4-6: Distribution of serum ferritin levels

Transferrin saturation was not recorded for all patients and was not a routinely performed laboratory parameter. Values were available for 245 patients. Mean transferrin saturation was 31 ± 15%. At baseline and month 6, transferrin saturation was 31 ± 15% (95 % CI: 29-33 %) and 30 ± 14% (95% CI: 28-31 %), respectively. 68% of the patients (n= 232 patients) received in addition to the epoetin therapy anti-anaemic medication, whereof 189 patients were given iron intravenously and 19 patients received oral iron substitution (24 patients were not specified). Two patients received blood transfusion before and at survey entry. Haemoglobin concentration of these two patients rose from 8.6 g/dl (before survey entry) to 9.8 g/dl (baseline) and from 7.3 g/dl (before study entry) to 9.3 g/dl (baseline).

Patients were classified into three categories according to their overall mean serum ferritin level (category 1= deficiency of serum ferritin: <100 µg/l; category 2= adequate serum ferritin: between ≥100 and <200 µg/l and category 3= optimal serum ferritin: ≥200 µg/l). Mean epoetin dose and mean haemoglobin level was calculated for each serum ferritin group. Mean baseline epoetin dose was significantly higher in the patient group with inadequate serum ferritin levels (190 ± 119 IU/kg/week) compared to the patient group with adequate iron stores (130 ± 74 IU/kg/week) (p value: 0.0039; Kruskal-Wallis test) and optimal iron stores (141 ± 110 IU/kg/week) (p value: 0.009; Kruskal-Wallis test). Baseline haemoglobin was lower in the group with inadequate serum ferritin levels compared to the patient groups with adequate (p value: 0.007 Kruskal-Wallis test) and optimal serum ferritin levels (p value: 0.0012; Kruskal-Wallis test). Patients with optimal iron status achieved higher haemoglobin levels compared to patients with iron deficiency at baseline. No significant difference was observed for epoetin dose and haemoglobin concentration between the three iron categories at month 6, as illustrated in Figure 4-12. Table 4-7 provides a more detailed overview with monthly epoetin doses and haemoglobin concentrations per group category of serum ferritin levels.

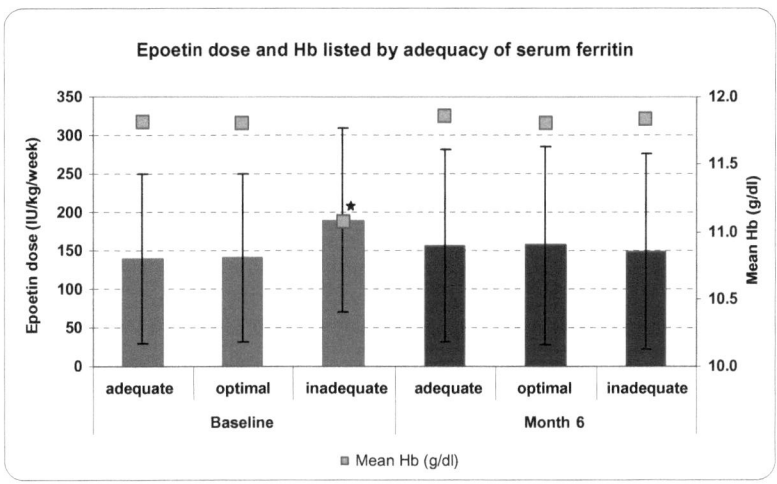

*significant difference for Hb and epoetin beta. No significance for month 6; Hb=haemoglobin concentration
inadequate: serum ferritin <100 µg/l; adequate: serum ferritin ≥100 µg/l <200 µg/l; optimal: serum ferritin ≥200 µg/l

Figure 4-12: Epoetin dose (±SD) and Hb (±SD) listed by serum ferritin at baseline and month 6

Visits	Group	Number of patients	Mean weekly epoetin dose (IU/kg/week) ± SD	Mean haemoglobin (g/dl) ± SD
Baseline	Adequate serum ferritin	39	130 ± 74	11.9 ± 1.6
	Optimal serum ferritin	275	141 ± 110	11.8 ± 1.4
	Inadequate serum ferritin	26	190 ± 119*	11.1 ± 1.6*
Month 1	Adequate serum ferritin	22	130 ± 86	12.0 ± 1.6
	Optimal serum ferritin	301	145 ± 108	11.7 ± 1.3
	Inadequate serum ferritin	17	120 ± 93	11.7 ± 1.3
Month 2	Adequate serum ferritin	27	133 ± 86	11.8 ± 1.7
	Optimal serum ferritin	289	155 ± 122	11.7 ± 1.4
	Inadequate serum ferritin	24	129 ± 89	11.8 ± 1.5
Month 3	Adequate serum ferritin	39	124 ± 80	12.0 ± 1.6
	Optimal serum ferritin	270	157 ± 126	11.8 ± 1.3
	Inadequate serum ferritin	31	133 ± 105	11.6 ± 1.4
Month 4	Adequate serum ferritin	44	111 ± 78**	12.2 ± 1.2[+]
	Optimal serum ferritin	264	160 ± 134	11.8 ± 1.2
	Inadequate serum ferritin	32	141 ± 107	11.5 ± 1.4
Month 5	Adequate serum ferritin	42	114 ± 85**	11.9 ± 1.3
	Optimal serum ferritin	265	159 ± 130	11.8 ± 1.3
	Inadequate serum ferritin	33	147 ± 111	11.9 ± 1.6
Month 6	Adequate serum ferritin	39	139 ± 104	12.2 ± 1.3
	Optimal serum ferritin	268	159 ± 128	11.8 ± 1.4
	Inadequate serum ferritin	33	148 ± 127	11.8 ± 1.6

*Significant difference observed at baseline between patients with inadequate serum ferritin and adequate iron stores ($p<0.05$ Kruskal-Wallis test) and with inadequate serum ferritin and optimal serum ferritin ($p<0.05$ Kruskal-Wallis test). **Significant difference between optimal serum ferritin and adeqate serum ferritin ($p= 0.02$ Kruskal-Wallis test).
[+]Significant difference between adequate and inadequate serum ferritin ($p=0.02$ Kruskal-Wallis test) and between adequate and optimal serum ferritin ($p=0.04$ Kruskal-Wallis test)

Table 4-7: Epoetin dose and haemoglobin listed by serum ferritin level

4.4.4 Inverse relationship between epoetin dose and haemoglobin

Our findings demonstrate an inverse relationship between mean haemoglobin and mean weekly epoetin dose, as illustrated in Figure 4-13. Mean weekly epoetin beta dose of patients with mean haemoglobin levels <11g/dl was 217 ± 146 IU/kg/week (95% CI: 183-252), and significantly higher compared to the mean weekly epoetin dose (132 ± 828 IU/kg/week; 95% CI: 122-142) of patients with mean haemoglobin levels ≥11 g/dl (p= 0.00001, Students' t-test). Serum ferritin of patients with mean haemoglobin <11 g/dl was 466 ± 393 µg/l and was comparable to the patients with mean haemoglobin <11 g/dl (426 ± 217 µg/l). Responses to epoetin treatment were comparable in women and in men. 19.2% of male patients and 21.8% of female patients had a haemoglobin level below 11 g/dl. The prevalence of patients with diabetes, coronary artery disease and heart failure did not occur more frequently in patients with lower haemoglobin levels (Hb <11 g/dl) than in patients with higher levels (p>0.1; χ^2-test). Comparable results were found in dialysis patients on maintenance phase (n=322 patients).

Non-responders and poor responders were classified according to different thresholds of mean weekly epoetin dose, i.e. ≥300 IU/kg/week (for non-response) and ≥200 IU/kg/week (for poor response), and were stratified by haemoglobin level. An inverse linear relationship was observed between the proportion of non-responders/poor responders and haemoglobin concentration (valid for Hb <12 g/dl).

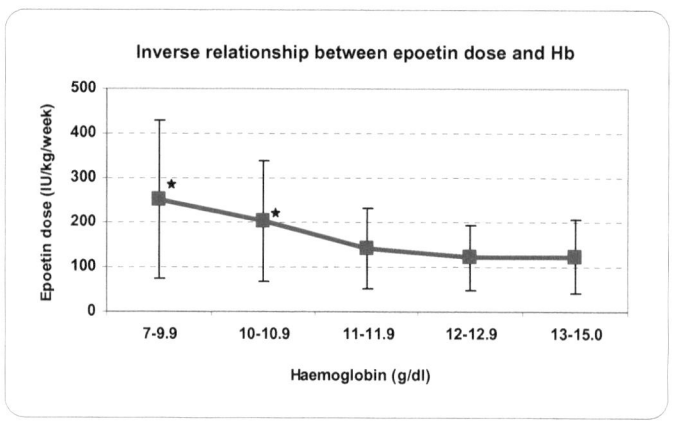

* significant difference

Figure 4-13: Inverse relation between epoetin dosage and haemoglobin (±SD)

Lower haemoglobin concentrations were associated with higher proportions of non- or poor responders, as illustrated in Figure 4-14. 33% of the patients at a haemoglobin level between 9-9.9g/dl (mean weekly epoetin dose ≥300 IU/kg) and 22% of the patients at a haemoglobin level between 10-10.9 g/dl, respectively, were non-responders. Comparable results were obtained in stable dialysis patients (n=322 patients), excluding epoetin-naïve patients (n=18 patients).

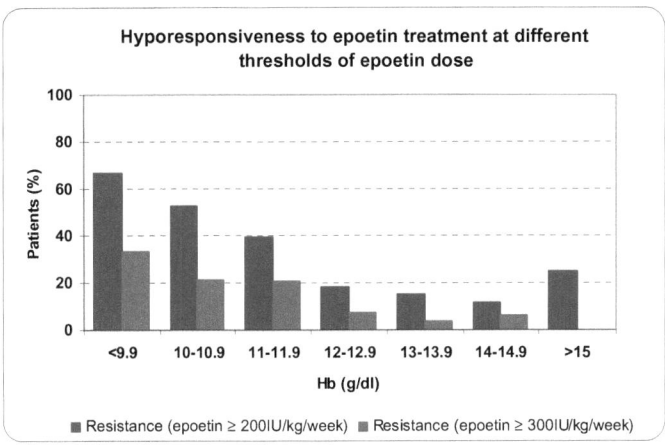

Figure 4-14: Hyporesponsiveness to epoetin treatment at mean weekly epoetin doses of 200 and 300 IU/kg/week

4.5 Discussion

The survey showed that anaemia was well controlled in dialysis patients in Switzerland. Haemoglobin level was on average above 11 g/dl for the majority of the patients. 90% of the patients had adequately replete iron stores (serum ferritin) and were in iron balance. Most patients required iron supplementation. In approximately 60% of the patients, epoetin beta was administered as 1x weekly dosing regimen and it was predominantly administered subcutaneously. Most patients were treated with mean weekly epoetin dosages below 10,000 IU/week; higher epoetin doses were required in approximately one fourth of the patients. Epoetin dose was shown to correlate negatively with haemoglobin concentration. Iron deficiency was found to be responsible for hyporesponsiveness to epoetin beta treatment at baseline.

Haemoglobin

Haemoglobin level remained stable during the six months observation period and no significant change in haemoglobin level was observed. In some studies, the assessed patients' parameters happen to improve during observation. Within this survey, however, only minor variations of haemoglobin concentration were observed, thus haemoglobin concentration remained stable for the majority of the patients. Improved haemoglobin concentrations were achieved in 4% of the patients.

Revised EBPG (edition 2004) recommend for dialysis patients a target haemoglobin level of ≥ 11g/dl [82]. In the "AIMS" survey, more than 70% of the patients achieved the recommended target haemoglobin level of 11 g/dl. Anaemia management fits for the majority of the dialysis patients into the recommendations of the EBPG [40]. Anaemia was well controlled in dialysis patients in Switzerland and a high quality of anaemia control was achieved. A higher proportion of dialysis patients in "AIMS" achieved the recommended target haemoglobin level compared to the findings of the "ESAM" survey, where 49% of the observed patients achieved the target level (baseline). Anaemia management of dialysis patients in Switzerland was above the European average (11.4 g/dl) and has obviously improved towards higher haemoglobin levels over the last half decade [119].

Anaemia treatment was comparable in male and female dialysis patients. Males were slightly on a higher haemoglobin level (11.9 g/dl) than females (11.7 g/dl). This difference in haemoglobin level between genders was greater in the age group between 31-40 years and decreased with increasing age. The difference is explainable by physiological reasons; menstruating women generally have lower haemoglobin concentrations than men or non-menstruating women [131].

Treatment with epoetin beta

Mean epoetin beta dose was 143 IU/kg/week at baseline and remained stable throughout the observation. The majority of the patients required weekly epoetin dosages lower than 200 IU/kg/week in order to maintain target haemoglobin level. Approximately 40% of the patients required even smaller epoetin doses (<100 IU/kg/week). According to the EBPG, epoetin doses between 50-150 IU/kg/week are recommended at therapy initiation and median maintenance dose given subcutaneously should normally be less than 125 IU/kg/week [40]. Median epoetin beta dose of patients in "AIMS" was 118 IU/kg/week and corresponded to the guidelines. Mean weekly epoetin beta dose, however, figured in the upper range of the recommendations. This can be explained by the fact that elevated haemoglobin concentrations result in higher epoetin dose requirements. Similar findings were found in other surveys as well.

Epoetin beta can be administered by different route of administration. The majority of the patients included in "AIMS" received epoetin beta subcutaneously with no significant change during the observation period. The subcutaneous administration of epoetin allows a 20-30% dose reduction compared to the intravenous administration. For economical reasons, the predominant route of administration had been subcutaneous for all recombinant erythropoietin products [73, 74]. For safety concerns, the subcutaneous administration of epoetin alfa was contraindicated in December 2002 by the European regulatory authorities. These safety restrictions did not concern epoetin beta. Nevertheless, a shift from the subcutaneous to intravenous administration was also expected for epoetin beta. A possible change in the route of administration would have been observed during the survey, since the survey just started at the time of the upcoming safety issue. The proportion of patients treated with either the subcutaneous or intravenous route of administration remained, though, unchanged during the survey.

In contrast to the literature [73, 74], mean epoetin beta dose was comparable for subcutaneous and intravenous administration. Whereas no difference in epoetin beta dose between the two routes of administration was observed, mean haemoglobin level was significantly lower in patients receiving epoetin beta intravenously compared to subcutaneous epoetin beta administration. Even though the survey was not designed to answer this question, our findings confirm a possible difference in the efficacy between the subcutaneous and intravenous route of administration with a tendency in favour of the subcutaneous administration of epoetin beta. 1x weekly administration of epoetin beta was the predominent dosing regimen in most Swiss dialysis centres when appropriate. Epoetin beta can be administered in different routes of administration and dosing frequencies according to the specific needs of patients, allowing individualized anaemia therapy for chronic kidney disease patients.

Iron

Iron is a relevant factor for the effectivity of erythropoiesis-stimulating treatments (ESAs) since a synergistic effect between iron and ESA therapy exists [105, 132]. In case of iron deficiency, unmatured reticulocytes will leave the bone marrow and, as a result, decrease haemoglobin concentration. Serum ferritin is the best available marker to assess iron store. Iron availability can be either assessed by means of the percentage of circulating hypochromic red cells or transferrin saturation.

Serum ferritin was well controlled in the majority of the patients. Half of those were within the optimal range of 200-500 µg/l recommended by the EBPG [40, 82]. Less than 10% of the patients had serum ferritin levels lower than the requested threshold of 100 µg/l, which is recommended for an adequate response to ESA therapy. Mean serum ferritin was comparable in female and in male patients. Transferrin saturation was not measured for all patients. Mean transferrin saturation of available measurements met the recommended target level for transferrin saturation. Most dialysis patients receive oral or parenteral iron therapy beside ESA treatment. Orally administered iron may be sufficient in the early stages of chronic kidney disease; parenteral iron substitution may become necessary in advanced chronic kidney disease. Studies showed that parenteral iron therapy improved haemoglobin level and allowed dose reduction of ESAs compared to orally administered iron [133-135]. Approximately 70% of the patients received additional anaemia treatment beside epoetin beta. Where documented, more than 80% of these were treated with parenteral iron therapy. The proportion of patients receiving iron substitution (oral and parenteral) may be underreported in this survey, but the results indicate that most patients on therapy with ESAs receive iron substitution in order to achieve target haemoglobin level.

Inverse relationship between haemoglobin and epoetin beta dose

An inverse relationship was found for epoetin beta dose and haemoglobin. Patients with lower haemoglobin level required significantly higher epoetin dose. The EBPG define resistance to epoetin treatment if epoetin dose of ≥300 IU/kg/week are used in order to achieve target haemoglobin level. Other definitions use a threshold of ≥200 IU/kg/week to classify poor response [119]. Using these cut-off levels, significantly more poor- and non-responders to epoetin beta were found at lower haemoglobin levels (Hb <11 g/dl). Haemoglobin levels of those patients were found to be significantly lower compared to responders.

One of the major reasons of hyporesponsiveness to epoetin treatment is iron deficiency [82]. Patients with chronic kidney disease should be in iron balance in order to maintain a haemoglobin concentration of at least 11 g/dl. To achieve this target haemoglobin, serum ferritin level should exceed 100 µg/l and transferrin saturation 20% [40, 82]. In our survey, mean serum ferritin was comparable between patients with lower (<11 g/dl; serum ferritin: 468 µg/l) and patients with higher haemoglobin levels (≥11 g/dl; serum ferritin: 430 µg/l). However, inadequate serum ferritin levels were associated with lower haemoglobin levels and higher epoetin dose requirements at baseline. This was not observed for month 1 to 6. Nevertheless, it indicates that repleted iron stores are an important factor for treatment response to ESAs. The reason why this association was only found at baseline was not conclusively explainable. In the next analysis, we will assess iron status according to the recommendations of current guidelines and its possible influence on resistance to epoetin treatment by inlcuding both iron markers, serum ferritin and transferrin saturation (see 5.4.5, page 89).

Beside iron deficiency, there are other reasons which might be responsible for hyporesponsiveness to ESA therapy. Several studies indicate that females predispose to an increased epoetin requirement and poorer response than male. This, however, was not found in our survey. Gender, age and co-morbidity did not occur more frequently in poor responders and were not found to be influencing factors. Some factors influencing the response to ESAs, such as inflammation and infection [136, 137], parathyroidism [138], concomitant medication (i.e. ACE inhibitor) have not been assessed within this survey and allow restricted conclusions on the causes of hyporesponsiveness regarding epoetin treatment. For further surveys in a comparable scope, we recommend the documentation of those parameters which may be associated with lower response to treatment with ESAs, such as C-reactive protein, which is a good indicator for inflammation, Kt/V (dialysis quality) and therapeutically relevant concomitant medication such as ACE inhibitor and AT_1 receptor blocker therapy [40, 82].

In conclusion, anaemia was well controlled and a high quality of anaemia control was achieved in the majority of the dialysis patients included in "AIMS". Anaemia treatment corresponded to the recommendations of the EBPG and is assessed in more detail in the following article (see section 5 page 75). Epoetin beta was predominantly administered as a 1x weekly dosing regimen, allowing more convenience for patients and health care people. Within the last five years, anaemia treatment improved towards higher haemoglobin levels [119], resulting in a better quality of anaemia control for dialysis patients in Switzerland. Many factors can influence the response to epoetin. Other factors, such as age, gender and inflammation can not be influenced. Iron management, however, can be controlled and is essential in order to achieve a high quality of anaemia treatment in dialysis patients. The present survey represents a simplified tool to perform quality assessments of anaemia management in chronic kidney disease patients, which can be easily implemented in each dialysis centre. It may also be valuable as a basis for the establishement of a Swiss national database for dialysis patients in order to improve patient care and facilitate individualized therapy.

5. Adherence of anaemia management in dialysis patients in Switzerland to the European Best Practice Guidelines (EBPG) for anaemia treatment in chronic kidney disease patients

N. Lötscher[1,2], D. Teta[3], D. Kiss[4], P.-Y. Martin[5], L. Gabutti[6], M. Burnier[3*]

1 Roche (Pharma) Switzerland Ltd, P.O. Box, CH-4153 Reinach, Switzerland
2 Swiss Tropical Institute, Department of Public Health and Epidemiology, P.O.Box, CH-4002 Basel, Switzerland
3 CHUV, Department of Internal Medicine, Nephrology, P.O. Box, CH-1011 Lausanne, Switzerland
4 Kantonsspital Liestal, Department of Nephrology, P.O. Box, CH-4410 Liestal, Switzerland
5 HCUG, Department of Internal Medicine, Nephrology, P.O. Box, CH-1211 Geneva, Switzerland
6 Ospedale regionale La Carità, Department of Nephrology, P.O. Box, CH-6601 Locarno, Switzerland

*Corresponding author:

Tel.:   +41 21 314 11 54
E-mail: michel.burnier@hospvd.ch

Working paper to be submitted

5.1 Abstract

Aim: The purpose of the second analysis of the survey "AIMS" (*Anaem*I*a* *M*anagement in dialysis patients in *S*witzerland) was to compare anaemia management in dialysis patients in Switzerland to the European Best Practice Guidelines for management of anaemia in patients with chronic renal failure (EBPG) and to assess potential differences between the clinical practice in Switzerland and the current guidelines. The second objective was to assess physicians' targets for anaemia treatment in Swiss dialysis centres.
Method: 368 dialyzed patients of 28 dialysis centres in Switzerland were included in this practice-based survey, 340 thereof were eligible. Anaemia treatment with epoetin beta in clinical practice was observed for 12 months and compared to the recommendations of the EBPG. Physicians' targets for anaemia treatment were assessed in respect of the guidelines and of the achieved values.
Results: Six months results were analyzed and compared to current guidelines. 79% of the patients achieved mean haemoglobin levels of ≥11 g/dl as recommended by the EBPG and 43% achieved mean haemoglobin levels of ≥12 g/dl. Physicians' targets for haemoglobin concentration were ≥11 g/dl and ranged between 11 and 13.5 g/dl. 58% of the centres aimed at a target haemoglobin level of ≥12 g/dl. 90% of the patients achieved adequate and 80% optimal targets for serum ferritin, which corresponded to the recommendations of the EBPG. Transferrin saturation was not a routinely performed laboratory parameter. Administered mean weekly epoetin beta dose was 149 ± 104 IU/kg/week (median: 122 IU/kg/week) and figured in the upper range of the recommendations. In contrast to the recommendation, epoetin beta was administered 1x weekly in the majority of epoetin-naïve patients at treatment initiation.
Conclusions: Anaemia management was well controlled in dialysis patients in Switzerland and most patients fit into the recommendations of the EBPG. Physicians' target haemoglobin was higher than the recommended target of the current guidelines. Administered epoetin dose was in the upper range of the recommendations resulting in elevated haemoglobin levels. Thus, a high quality of anaemia therapy of dialysis patients was achieved in Swiss dialysis centres which improved reaching higher haemoglobin targets over the recent years.

Key words: Anaemia, anaemia management, epoetin, epoetin beta, dosing frequency, end-stage renal disease, European Best Practice Guidelines

5.2 Introduction

The survey *Anaem*I*a Management in dialysis patients in* S*witzerland* "AIMS" was conducted from June 2002 and ended at December 2004. Patient inclusion lasted from June 2002 until December 2003 with an observation period of 12 months. It was the first large-scale survey in Switzerland, after the edition of the EBPG, assessing the quality of anaemia treatment in dialysis patients in Switzerland over a time period of 12 months. In the first analysis (see section 4, page 54), we assessed the quality of the anaemia control in dialysis patients in Switzerland. The findings of the first analysis showed that anaemia was well controlled in the majority of the dialysis patients cared in Swiss dialysis centres. Approximately 80% of the patients achieved a haemoglobin concentration of ≥11g/dl and more than 40% a haemoglobin concentration of ≥12g/dl. Mean haemoglobin level increased towards 12 g/dl over the recent years improving from 11.4 g/dl in 1998 (results of "ESAM") [119]) to 11.8 g/dl achieved in this survey. Anaemia treatment and the efficacy of anaemia therapy were monthly monitored in all patients included in "AIMS" and adapted if required. This regular and careful monitoring of anaemia treatment in Swiss dialysis centres may have contributed to achieve a high quality of anaemia management in these patients. In the second analysis, the findings of the current anaemia management of dialysis patients in Switzerland were compared with the current guidelines for the management of anaemia in patients with chronic renal failure and are presented in this article [40, 82].

The first guidelines were published in 1996 by the US National Kidney Foundation-Dialysis Outcome Quality Initiative (NKF-DOQI), based on a critical review of 2836 published papers. Although NKF-DOQI guidelines were available, there was a need for recommendations reflecting current European clinical practice and experience. A group of representative experts of the ERA-EDTA and the societies of nephrology of the European Union, Central and Eastern European countries published the "European Best Practice Guidelines for the management of anaemia in patients with chronic renal failure (EBPG) in 1999 in adherence to the NKF-DOQI guidelines. In 2004, revised guidelines had been published to address changes in the field of anaemia management, such as new erythropoietic agents, adverse events and discussions on the appropriate target haemoglobin. The publication of the EBPG was the first important step in process; however, their implementation in clinical practice is even more important. The guidelines recommend target haemoglobin levels greater than 11 g/dl in the management of anaemia in dialysis patients. Current practice of anaemia correction aims at partial normalization of anaemia. The European Survey in Anaemia Management (ESAM) gave evidence that even these modest targets postulated by the EBPG for anaemia treatment were not achieved [119]. The risk-benefit ratio of the optimum target above this level has not been established and remains still unclear. There is an association between low haemoglobin concentrations and cardiovascular disease in chronic kidney disease patients, suggesting that normalization of haemoglobin concentration may be appropriate [3, 31, 120, 121]. However, the US Normal Hematocrit Study showed a higher incidence of death or non-fatal myocardial infarction in the group with higher haematocrit levels than in the one with lower levels [115]. These results were unexpected and might have influenced physicians' behaviour regarding anaemia treatment in dialysis patients.

EBPG recommendations	Target	Comment
Haemoglobin	≥11 g/dl	Target Hb ≥11 g/dl, individually defined (range: 11-14 g/dl) in respect of gender, age, activity and co-morbid conditions
		Hb concentrations >12 g/dl are not recommended for CHF and diabetes
Iron	Serum ferritin: ≥100 µg/l TsF: ≥20%	Optimum serum ferritin: 200-500 µg/l, TsF: 30-40% Upper limit for serum ferritin: 800 µg/l
Starting with ESA	Start: Hb <11 g/dl Hb response: 1-2 g/dl/month	Change to <1 g/dl: Total weekly ESA dose adjustment stepwise by 25%
Dosing of epoetin*	Epoetin: 50-150 IU/kg/week	Typically 4,000-8,000 IU/week Median maintenance dose: <125 IU/kg/week, with 90% of the patients receiving <300 IU/kg/week
Resistance	Epoetin >300 IU/kg/week Darbepoetin >1.5 µg/kg/week	Resistance is suspected when patient fails to attain the target Hb while receiving ESA doses higher than 300 IU/kg/week or 1.5 µg/kg/week

*based on EBPG (1998)
CHF=congestive heart failue; Route of administration and dosing frequency can be looked up in Table 1-5, page 29

Table 5-1: Overview of targets recommended by the EBPG in anaemia treatment

Thus, in the second analysis we compared the anaemia management in Switzerland with the recommendations of the EBPG in order to assess discrepancies in the application of the recommendations in everyday clinical practice. The second objective was to assess physicians' targets for anaemia management in respect of the guidelines and of the achieved values. The targets recommended by the EBPG for anaemia treatment are summarized in the outline above (Table 5-1).

5.3 Subjects and methods

Patients and data collection

"AIMS" was a prospective practice-based, open intervention survey designed to examine anaemia management in haemodialysis and peritoneal dialysis patients in Switzerland. 368 dialysis patients of 28 Swiss dialysis centres were included in this survey, whereof 340 of 26 centres were eligible. Inclusion and exclusion criteria were defined in more detail earlier, i.e. section 3.2, page 37. In brief, included patients were dialysis patients with renal anaemia, either pre-treated with epoetin or epoetin-naïve patients. Exclusion criteria were defined for patients with unstable angina pectoris, untreated hypertension, haemoglobinopathy, pregnancy, lactation, iron or vitamin B_{12} deficiencies. At survey initiation, baseline parameters of each patient, such as demographics, medical history, primary causes of chronic renal failure, concomitant diseases and current anaemia treatment were collected.

The aim of this survey was to document current anaemia management with epoetin beta in dialysis patients for 12 months. Therefore, anaemia treatment of dialysis patients (haemoglobin, iron status and epoetin beta dose) was monthly assessed over a time period of 12 months. No interference in anaemia treatment was required. Laboratory parameters were documented if performed in the course of the clinical routine. The schedule of assessments provides a closer overview of the survey procedure and is illustrated in Table 5-2. For more detailed information about survey aim, subjects and methods of "AIMS", see section 3, page 36.

The primary objective of this second analysis was to assess anaemia management in dialysis patients treated in Swiss dialysis centres and to compare the achievements with the recommendations of the EBPG [40, 82]. Achieved haemoglobin levels and iron stores were analysed in respect of the recommended targets in Section II of the EBPG (previously guidelines 5-6) and epoetin treatment, i.e., epoetin dose, route of administration and administration frequency were compared to the recommendations in Section III of the EBPG (previously guidelines 9-12). A short outline of the recommended targets by the EBPG is given in Table 5-1.

The second objective consisted in assessing, centre-specific targets for anaemia treatment in dialysis patients in Switzerland. For this purpose, a questionnaire was sent to all participating dialysis centres asking them to report their specific targets in anaemia treatment of dialysis patients. Target values for haemoglobin, serum ferritin and transferrin saturation were documented by each participating dialysis centre. Individual centre-specific targets were then compared to the achieved values in "AIMS" and to the recommendations of the EBPG.

Schedule of assessments	Baseline	Monthly reports (M1–M12)	Final report (M12 or study interruption)
Medical history	x		
Weight	x	x	
Blood pressure	x		
Epoetin treatment	x		
Concomitant anaemia treatment	x	x	
Epoetin beta dose/frequency	x	x	
Route of administration	x	x	
Adverse events		x	
Laboratory data			
– haemoglobin	x	x	
– transferrin saturation	x	x	
– ferritin*	x	x	
– creatinine*	x	x	
Assessment of efficacy and practicability	x	x	x

*where available

Table 5-2: Schedule of assessments

Statistical analysis

All patients who received at least one treatment of epoetin beta after patient registration were included in the analysis. Patients were excluded from the survey according to the inclusion and exclusion criteria. Missing values were replaced by using the last observation carried forward method (LOCF). Simple statistics were performed in Excel 2002 or Epi-Info®, version 3.2. Complex statistics were performed using the SAS statistical program version 8.2 (SAS, Institute, Cary, NC, USA). Standard descriptive statistics (mean, median, standard deviation [SD], and confidence interval [CI]) were calculated for all study variables, such as haemoglobin, epoetin dose, administration frequency, route of administration, serum ferritin and transferrin saturation. Categorical variables were compared using the χ^2-test and continuous variables using Students' t-test, Wilcoxon two-sample and Kruskal-Wallis test where appropriate. All statistical tests were two-sided and the significance was tested on a 0.05 p value.

5.4 Results

Six month data are presented in this article. The analysis was performed on 340 eligible dialysis patients. 28 patients were excluded from the study due to missing efficacy parameters for all six months. Section 3.8.1, page 47 provides a closer overview of patient exclusion and the remaining treatment population.

5.4.1 Patient characteristics

The age distribution of patients included in "AIMS" ranged from 18-91, with a mean age of 63.5 ± 14.7 and a median of 67 years. 142 of the eligible patients were female (42%) and 198 patients were male (58%). 324 patients were on haemodialysis and 16 on peritoneal dialysis. Patient characteristics, concomitant diseases and diagnosis of chronic kidney disease are described earlier in section 3.8.2, page 47. In brief, the most common causes of end-stage renal failure were glomerulonephritis (23.2%), diabetic nephropathy

(20.9%), hypertension and vascular diseases (21.2%). Table 5-3 provides a closer overview of diagnosis of end-stage renal disease in patients in "AIMS". Most frequent concomitant diseases were hypertension (60.6%), coronary artery disease (25.5%), diabetes (27.4%) and congestive heart failure (16.5%). Less frequent concomitant diseases were vascular diseases (5%), metabolic disorders (2%), hepatological disorders (2%), cancer (2%) and pulmonary diseases (COPD) (1.8%). Mean baseline blood pressure was 161 ± 23 mmHg and 86 ± 16 mmHg. Of the 340 dialysis patients included in "AIMS", 94.7 % were pre-treated with epoetin (n=322 patients) and 5.3% were epoetin-naïve patients (n=18 patients). Baseline haemoglobin level was 11.8 ± 1.4 g/dl and serum ferritin 411± 297 µg/l.

Diagnosis	n	%	Mean age ± SD
Diabetic nephropathy	71	20.9	64.2 ± 11.7
Glomerulonephritis	79	23.2	59.4 ± 14.7
Pyelonephritis / interstitial nephritis	58	17.1	62.9 ± 13.5
Hypertension / vascular causes	72	21.2	69.0 ± 12.4
Polycystic kidney disease	27	7.9	59.4 ±15.6
Neoplasm / tumours	9	2.6	67.3 ± 11.2
Unclear	13	3.8	62.7 ± 16.8
Miscellaneous causes	10	2.9	55.6 ± 23.2
Missing	9	2.6	62.2 ± 19.2

Multiple entries possible, therefore not cumulative

Table 5-3: Diagnosis of end-stage renal disease (ESRD) in "AIMS"

5.4.2 Haemoglobin targets for anaemia treatment

Recommendations for haemoglobin targets by the EBPG

Mean haemoglobin at baseline was 11.8 ± 1.4 g/dl, ranging from 6.8 to 15.5 g/dl (95% CI: 11.6-11.9 g/dl). Overall, mean haemoglobin was 11.8 ± 1.0 g/dl, and median value of haemoglobin was 11.9 g/dl. 79 % of the patients achieved mean haemoglobin levels of ≥11 g/dl, as recommended by the European Best Practice Guidelines and illustrated in Figure 5-1. 43% of the patients were at a mean haemoglobin level of ≥12 g/dl. Mean haemoglobin levels were 11.8 ± 1.0 g/dl for patients on haemodialysis (n=323) and ranged from 8.4 to 14.3 g/dl. For peritoneal dialysis patients (n=17), mean haemoglobin concentrations were 11.6 ± 1.0 g/dl and ranged from 8.8 g/dl to 14.6 g/dl. 80% (n=257 of 323) of the haemodialysis patients achieved haemoglobin levels of ≥11g/dl and 43% haemoglobin levels of ≥12 g/dl. Similar results were obtained in patients on peritoneal dialysis. 77% and 41% of peritoneal dialysis patients achieved target haemoglobin levels of ≥11 g/dl and ≥12 g/dl, respectively.

Centre-specific targets for haemoglobin

Mean haemoglobin concentration was in 95% of the dialysis centres higher than the haemoglobin target of ≥11 g/dl recommended by the EBPG. Physicians' haemoglobin targets were in all dialysis centres above 11 g/dl and ranged between 11 and 13.5 g/dl. In 15 of 26 dialysis centres (= 57.7% of the participating centres), physicians aimed at target haemoglobin levels ≥12 g/dl. 79% of all patients achieved 11g/dl as recommended by the guidelines; however, only 48% of the patients achieved their target haemoglobin concentration (see Figure 5-1).

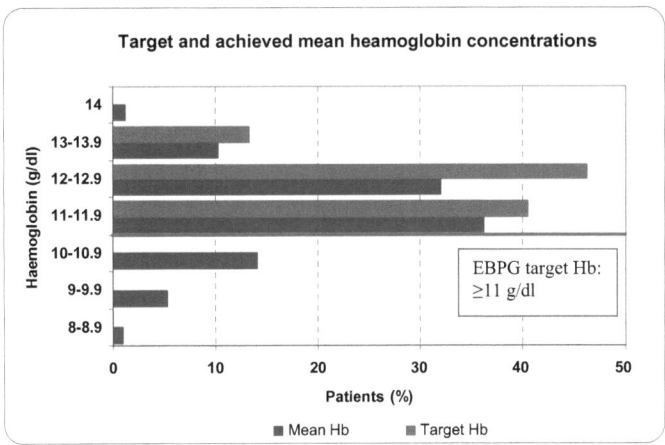

Figure 5-1: Distribution of physicians' target Hb and achieved mean Hb level over 6 months

If anaemia management in "AIMS" met the requirements of the EBPG the following conditions were expected: 1) target haemoglobin of at least 11 g/dl per patient; 2) the majority of co-ordinate points on a regression line between 11 and 13 g/dl and 3) the majority of co-ordinates to be distributed in the upper right sector of the graph. Figure 5-2 shows the association between physicians' target haemoglobin levels and achieved levels.

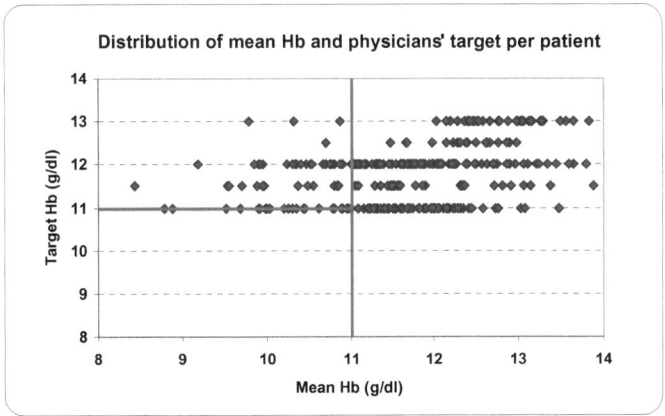

Figure 5-2: Distribution of achieved mean Hb and physicians' target Hb

79% of the patients were distributed in the upper right and corresponded at least to the recommendations of the EBPG. Physicians' target haemoglobin levels were achieved in approximately half of the patients (163 patients), since in the majority of the centres the physiccians' targets were higher than recommended by EBPG.

Figure 5-3 illustrates the proportion of patients with achieved physicians' target per dialysis centre and physicians' target levels. In most dialysis centres physicians' target haemoglobin levels were higher than the target haemoglobin level recommended by the guidelines.

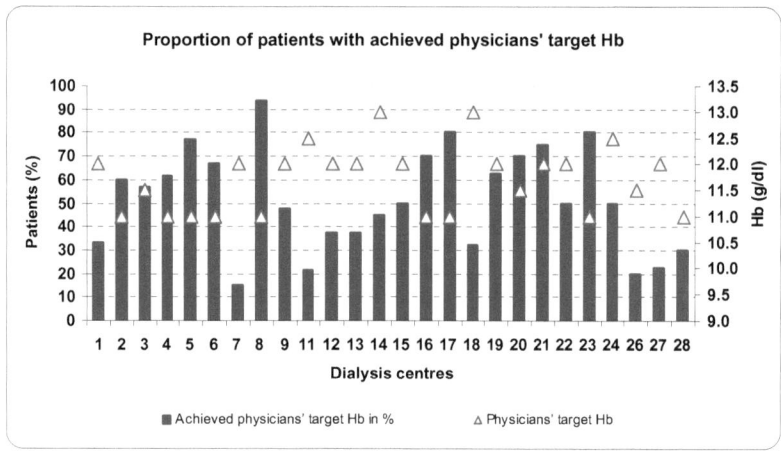

Figure 5-3: Proportion of dialysis patients with achieved physicians' target haemoglobin level

In centres where physicians' target haemoglobin level was 11 g/dl, 60 to 80% of the dialysis patients achieved the target. The proportion of patients achieving physicians' target haemoglobin was smaller in dialysis centres aiming at higher targets such as 12 and 13 g/dl. The response rate in these centres ranged from 14% (dialysis centre 7) at the lowest and 75% (dialysis centre 21) at the highest. Physicians' target haemoglobin was achieved in 16 dialysis centres (=61.5%) Whereas the target haemoglobin level recommended by the EBPG was achieved in 90% of all participating dialysis centres, fewer dialysis centres achieved their centre-specific target for haemoglobin.

Table 5-4 shows the physicians' target haemoglobin levels and achieved mean haemoglobin concentrations listed by the participating dialysis centre.

Dialysis centre	Number of patients	Achieved mean Hb g/dl	Physicians' target Hb g/dl (Hct: %)
1	3	11.3	12
2	5	10.9	11.5-12.5
3	23	11.7	11-12
4	26	11.0	11-12
5	13	11.5	>11
6	6	12.6	12
7	34	11.3	12
8	16	12.2	11-12
9	19	12.1	12
11	14	12.0	12.5
12	16	11.4	12
13	16	11.8	12
14	20	12.6	13 (40)
15	2	12.0	12
16	10	11.5	11-12
17	5	11.5	11-13 (33-36)
18	25	12.8	13
19	8	12.2	12-13
20	10	11.9	>11.5
21	4	13.0	12
22	14	12.1	12-13
23	10	11.4	11-12
24	12	12.6	12.5-13.5
26	10	10.5	11.5
27	9	11.8	12
28	10	10.9	11-12

No values for centre 10 and 25 due to study exclusion (missing reports). Hct=haematocrit

Table 5-4: Overview of achieved mean haemoglobin and centre-specific target haemoglobin levels

5.4.3 Iron targets for anaemia treatment

Recommendations for iron targets by the EBPG

92% and 89% of the patients presented with adequate iron stores with a mean serum ferritin of ≥100 µg/l at baseline and at month 6, as recommended by the EBPG. The percentage of patients with inadequate serum ferritin ranged concentration from 5-9.7% at any time during the observation period. Serum ferritin ranged within the recommended target levels of 200 and 500 µg/l (optimal replete iron stores) in 64% and exceeded the recommended upper limit of 800 µg/l in 8.5% of the patients in "AIMS". In 4.4% of the patients, serum ferritin levels were higher than 1,000 µg/l. The distribution of mean serum ferritin levels was analysed in haemodialysis and peritoneal dialysis patients. Adequate target serum ferritin (≥100 µg/l) was achieved in all peritoneal dialysis patients and in 97% of the haemodialysis patients. Optimal target serum ferritin (≥200 µg/l) was achieved in 88% of the haemodialysis and in 94% of the peritoneal dialysis patients (see Figure 5-4).

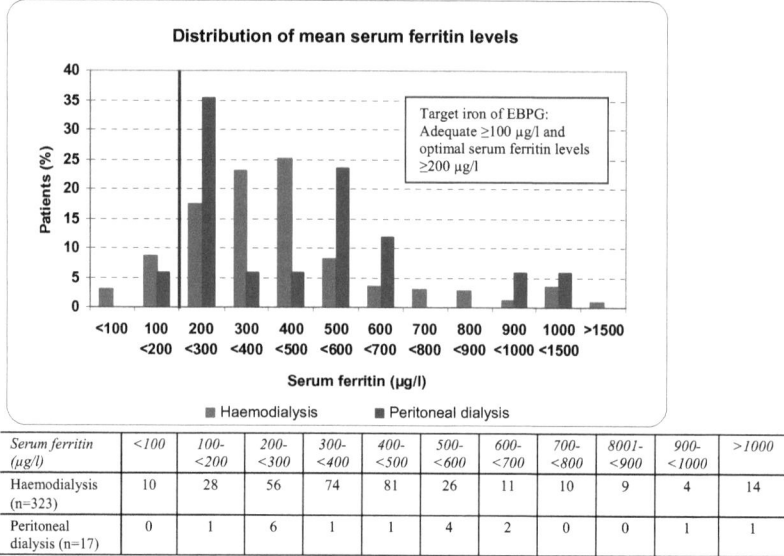

Serum ferritin (µg/l)	<100	100-<200	200-<300	300-<400	400-<500	500-<600	600-<700	700-<800	8001-<900	900-<1000	>1000
Haemodialysis (n=323)	10	28	56	74	81	26	11	10	9	4	14
Peritoneal dialysis (n=17)	0	1	6	1	1	4	2	0	0	1	1

Figure 5-4: Distribution of mean serum ferritin levels listed by dialysis treatment

Transferrin saturation was not measured for all patients, as it was a routinely measured laboratory parameter in all participating Swiss dialysis centres. Data were available for 245 of 340 patients at month 6. Mean transferrin saturation was 31 ± 13% and within the recommended optimal target range of 30-40%. Figure 5-5 illustrates the proportion of patients achieving EBPG targets for transferrin saturation.

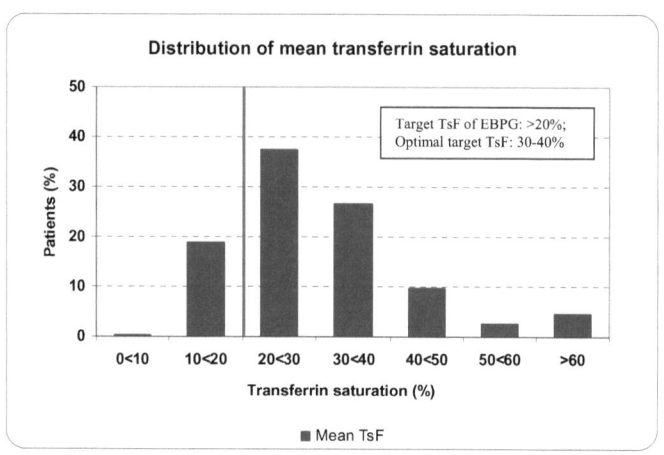

Figure 5-5: Distribution of mean transferrin saturation

80% of the patients achieved the minimum recommended transferrin saturation of 20%. 20% of the patients showed inadequate transferrin saturation values. Optimal target levels of 30% were achieved in 42% of the patients. Patients with available transferrin saturation values were classified according to their iron status into the following three different categories: absolute iron deficiency (serum ferritin <100 µg/l), functional iron deficiency (serum ferritin ≥100 µg/l and transferrin saturation <20%) and adequate iron status (serum ferritin levels ≥100 µg/l and transferrin saturation ≥20%). Adequate iron status: ≥100 µg/l and TsF ≥20%; functional iron deficiency: ≥100 µg/l and TsF <20%; absolute iron deficiency <100 µg/l.

Table 5-5 illustrates the prevalence of patients with iron deficiency and adequate iron stores. Adequate iron status was achieved in 67-71% of the patients throughout the survey.

Iron status	Total number of patients (%)	Adequate iron status Patients (%)	Functional iron deficiency Patients (%)	Absolute iron deficiency Patients (%)
Baseline	186 (54.7)	132 (71.0)	28 (15.1)	26 (14.0)
Month 1	215 (63.2)	153 (71.2)	45 (20.9)	17 (7.9)
Month 2	242 (71.2)	171 (70.7)	47 (19.4)	24 (9.9)
Month 3	253 (74.4)	176 (69.6)	46 (18.2)	31 (12.3)
Month 4	253 (74.4)	169 (66.8)	52 (20.6)	32 (12.6)
Month 5	257 (75.6)	177 (68.9)	47 (18.3)	33 (12.8)
Month 6	256 (75.3)	171 (66.8)	52 (20.3)	33 (12.9)

Adequate iron status: ≥100 µg/l and TsF ≥20%; Functional iron deficiency: ≥100 µg/l and TsF <20%; Absolute iron deficiency <100µg/l

Table 5-5: Distribution of patients according to iron status

Centre-specific targets for iron

Physicians' targets for serum ferritin were in the majority of the dialysis centres higher than the recommended target of 200 µg/l by the EBPG. Half of the centres followed the recommendation of the EBPG and aimed at optimum serum ferritin levels between 200 and 500 µg/l. One third of the centres did not define upper limits for serum ferritin. EBPG guidelines, however, recommend an upper limit of 800 µg/l for serum ferritin. 70% of all patients (n=240) achieved physicians' target for serum ferritin. Serum ferritin was regularly measured in all centres. In contrast, transferrin saturation was in one third of the centres not or only occasionally measured. Physicians' targets for transferrin saturation ranged from 20% (lowest; n=8) to 40% (highest; n=2). 15 of 18 centres measured for transferrin achieved their centre-specific target levels. More details are provided in Table 5-6.

Centre	Patients (n)	Achieved mean serum ferritin (µg/l)	Target serum ferritin (µg/l)	Achieved mean TsF (%) (patients)	Target TsF (%)	Comment
1	3	789	300-500	25 (3)	-	Not regularly measured
2	5	338	>200	30 (5)	>20	
3	23	399	300-500	26 (20)	>20	
4	26	352	>200	30 (1)	-	TsF not regularly measured
5	13	450	200-500	28 (13)	30-40	Target TsF not defined
6	6	199	>200	21 (5)	>20	
7	34	468	300-500	42 (8)	-	Not routinely measured
8	16	448	400-600	41 (16)	>20	
9	19	387	<400	36 (18)	30	
11	14	486	<600	25 (14)	>20	
12	16	726	400-600	-	20	
13	16	573	200-400	28 (16)	20-30	Measured if no iron administration
14	20	440	200	33 (20)	25	
15	2	400	>150	-	>20	
16	10	276	200-400	30 (10)	>20	Not regularly measured
17	5	277	<800	31 (5)	>25	
18	25	406	200-500	30 (25)	25	
19	8	709	>150 -600	38 (4)	-	Not measured
20	10	332	>200	23 (6)	-	
21	4	551	200-500	30 (4)	25-35	
22	14	414	200-500	29 (14)	20-40	
23	10	345	>300	9 (1)	-	Not regularly measured
24	12	300	>200 - <1000	29 (12)	20-30	
26	10	305	>200	26 (10)	>20	
27	9	475	>150	45 (8)	-	Rarely measured
28	10	363	>200	-	-	Not measured

TsF= transferrin saturation in %. No values for centre 10 and 25 due to survey exclusion (missing reports). In brackets, number of patients

Table 5-6: Achieved and target serum ferritin and transferrin levels per dialysis centre

5.4.4 Targets for treatment of renal anaemia with ESAs

Route of administration and dosing frequency of epoetin beta

In the "AIMS" survey, 69% of the patients received epoetin beta subcutaneously and 31% intravenously (at month 6). 65% of the intravenously treated patients received epoetin beta as a 1x weekly dosing regimen, even though there is lack of evidence to support 1x weekly dosing of intravenous epoetin in dialysis patients. 90% of the epoetin-naïve patients (16 of 18 patients) received epoetin beta as a 1x weekly dosing regimen already at treatment initiation, whereof 4 patients received epoetin beta intravenously. 67% of the stable patients in maintenance phase (pre-treated, n=322) received epoetin beta as a 1x weekly dosing regimen at baseline.

Treatment initiation with epoetin beta

18 of 340 patients were epoetin-naïve patients with treatment initiation at baseline. Epoetin beta dose and haemoglobin concentrations were compared between epoetin-pre-treated (n=322) and epoetin-naïve patients (n=18). Mean epoetin dose was 178 ± 165

IU/kg/week for epoetin-naïve patients and 148 ± 102 IU/kg/week for patients pre-treated with epoetin, which resulted in a dose difference of 20%. Figure 5-6 illustrates the monthly administered epoetin dose and haemoglobin concentration of epoetin-naïve and epoetin-pre-treated patients for 6 months. At baseline and month 1, administered epoetin dose was comparable in both groups. An increase of epoetin dose by 34% occurred in epoetin-naïve patients at month 2, leading to a relevant increase of haemoglobin level. Steady state was achieved after 3 months of epoetin treatment and corresponded to the recommended 2 to 4 months duration of titration phase recommended by the EBPG in order to reach target haemoglobin. Epoetin dose was reduced at month 6 by approximately 10% compared to the previous dose at month 5. After 3 months of epoetin treatment, comparable haemoglobin concentrations were achieved in epoetin-naïve and patients pre-treated with epoetin (p=0.4664; Students' t-test). Significant differrences in haemoglobin concentrations between those patients occurred at baseline, month 1 and month 2 (baseline: p=0.0001; month 1: p=0.0048; month 2: p=0.0403; Students' t-test). Mean haemoglobin concentration in epoetin-naïve patients was 10.2 ± 1.9 g/dl at baseline, 10.7 ± 1.6 g/dl at month 1, 11.0 ± 1.8 g/dl at month 2, 11.5 ± 1.8 g/dl at month 3, 11.7 ± 1.5 g/dl at month 4, 11.7 ± 1.4 g/dl at month 5 and 12.0 ± 1.7 g/dl at month 6, respectively. Haemoglobin response was 0.4 g/dl between baseline and month 1 and 1.3 g/dl over a time period of 3 months. Response to epoetin was lower than recommended by the EBPG, which postulate an increase of haemoglobin of 1-2 g/dl per month. Mean weekly epoetin dose was significantly higher in epoetin-naïve patients at month 2-5 compared to pre-treated patients with epoetin (month 2: p=0.01; month 3: p=0.01; month 4: p=0.008; month 5: p=0.008; Students' t-test). No significant difference was observed for epoetin dose between groups at baseline, month 1 and month 6. Table 5-7 provides a detailed overview of epoetin beta dose and haemoglobin concentration in epoetin-naïve and patients pre-treated with epoetin.

Epoetin beta dose	IU/kg per/week	Baseline	Month 1	Month 2	Month 3	Month 4	Month 5	Month 6
Epoetin-naïve patients (n=18)	Mean	144.5	151.2	199.8	191.1	192.6	194.4	173.9
	SD	102.4	105.5	199.1	196.8	204.4	203.5	195.8
Epoetin-pre-treated patients (n=322)	Mean	143.3	142.3	148.2	149.1	150.2	150.0	154.4
	SD	108.1	106.0	110.7	114.1	121.1	118.1	120.8
Difference	%	0.8	6.2	34.8	28.1	28.2	29.6	12.6
p value		0.52	0.33	0.001	0.01	0.008	0.008	0.10

Haemoglobin	(g/dl)	Baseline	Month 1	Month 2	Month 3	Month 4	Month 5	Month 6
Epoetin-naïve patients (n=18)	Mean	10.23	10.65	11.02	11.49	11.65	11.73	11.98
	SD	1.85	1.60	1.82	1.79	1.50	1.37	1.26
Epoetin-pre-treated patients (n=322)	Mean	11.82	11.79	11.76	11.78	11.86	11.83	11.85
	SD	1.35	1.31	1.34	1.35	1.24	1.37	1.41
Difference	g/dl	1.59	1.14	0.74	0.29	0.21	0.10	-0.13
p value		0.0001	0.005	0.04	0.47	0.55	0.50	0.81

Table 5-7: Response to epoetin beta treatment in epoetin-naïve and epoetin-pre-treated patients

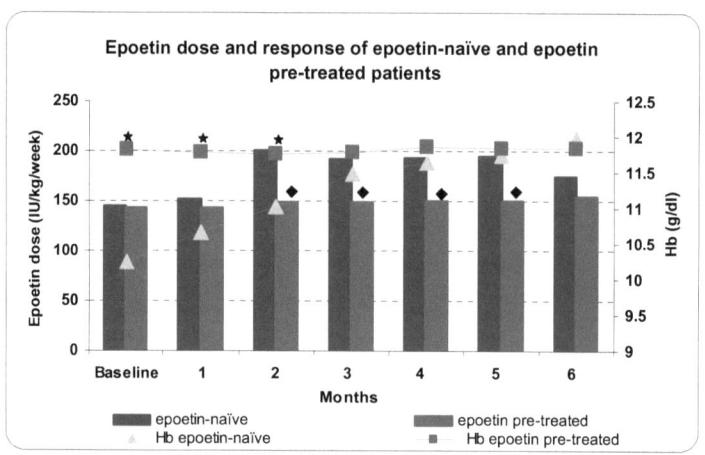

* Significance for haemoglobin; ♦ significance for epoetin dose

Figure 5-6: Epoetin beta dose and response of epoetin-naïve and epoetin pre-treated patients

Figure 5-7 reflects the haemoglobin distribution of epoetin-naïve patients (n=18 patients) at epoetin treatment initiation and after 6 months of epoetin beta treatment. At treatment initiation, two third of all epoetin-naïve patients had a haemoglobin level below 11 g/dl, one third of the patients had haemoglobin levels of 11 g/dl or higher and one patient showed a haemoglobin level >12 g/dl at epoetin treatment initiation. After 6 months of epoetin therapy, none of the patients' haemoglobin level was below 10 g/dl. 72% of the patients had haemoglobin levels of 11 g/dl or higher; in 61% of the patients, the levels were above 12 g/dl. Mean overall increase of haemoglobin level was 1.7 ± 2.5 g/dl (median: 2.4 g/dl) over 6 months. In patients with haemoglobin levels ≥11 g/dl at month 6, the mean increase of haemoglobin was 2.9 g/dl compared to baseline.

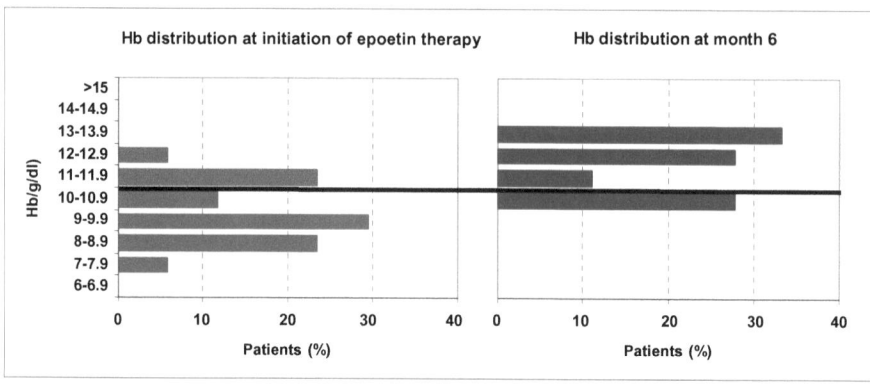

Figure 5-7: Initial Hb levels in epoetin-naïve patients and after 6 months of epoetin treatment

Dose response of stable dialysis patients with haemoglobin levels <11 g/dl

The development of the relationship of haemoglobin and epoetin dose after 6 months was analysed for stable patients on epoetin treatment with a baseline Hb <11g/dl and epoetin dose of <300 IU/kg/week. The distribution of the haemoglobin according to the epoetin dose at baseline and at month 6 is illustrated in Figure 5-8. Of 65 patients with a suboptimal response at baseline (Hb <11 g/dl, epoetin dose <300 IU/week), 26.2% and 55.3% achieved haemoglobin levels of ≥12 g/dl and ≥11 g/dl at month 6, respectively. Haemoglobin level of 44.6% of patients remained below 11 g/dl, 7.7% thereof having changed from a suboptimal response (<11g/dl, epoetin dose <300 IU/kg/week) to an inadequate response (<11g/dl, epoetin dose >300 IU/kg/week).

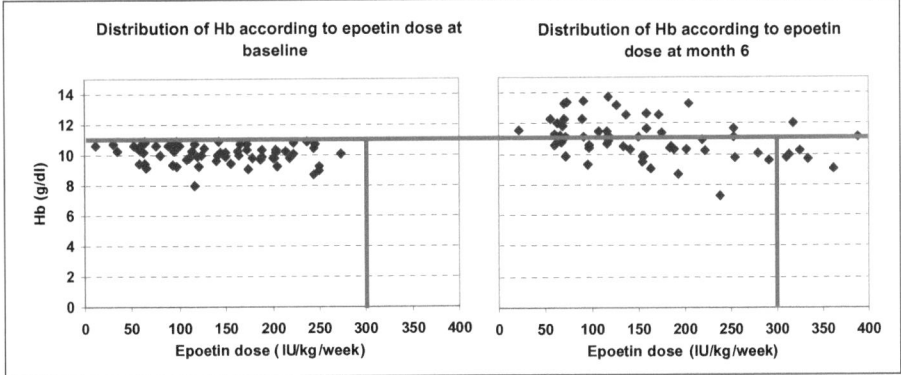

Figure 5-8: Change of relationship of Hb and epoetin dose after 6 months in patients with baseline Hb <11 g/dl and epoetin dose <300 IU/kg/week

5.4.5 Failure to respond to treatment

Mean epoetin beta dose of the total population in our survey was 149 ± 104 IU/kg/week (median: 122 IU/week). In 30 of 340 patients (8%), the administration of high epoetin dosages, defined as epoetin dose ≥300 IU/kg/week, was necessary in order to achieve or maintain target haemoglobin level. 12 of 30 patients requiring epoetin dose >300 IU/kg/week were found to be resistant to epoetin treatment (Hb <11 g/dl and epoetin dose >300IU/kg/week) according to the guidelines. Patients resistant to epoetin beta required significantly higher epoetin beta doses and achieved significantly lower haemoglobin concentrations than responding patients. Serum ferritin concentration was significantly higher in patient resistant to epoetin beta and ranged in the upper limit of the target serum ferritin recommended by the guidelines.

Median maintenance dose of stable dialysis patients responding to epoetin treatment, was 120 IU/kg/week and corresponded to the guidelines, which recommend a median maintenance dose of less than 125 IU/kg/week in more than 90% of the patients receiving <300 IU/kg/week (~ 20,000 IU/week).

Response to epoetin treatment	Non-responders	Responders	p value
Number of stable dialysis (n)	12	310	
Mean haemoglobin (g/dl) ± SD Confidence interval	10.4 ± 0.3 10.2–10.6	11.9 ± 1.0 10.9–12.0	<0.0001
Mean epoetin dose (IU/lkg/week) ± SD Confidence interval	454 ± 106 394–514	136 ± 82 55–145	<0.0001
Mean serum ferritin (µg/l) ± SD Confidence interval	740 ± 429 498–983	425 ±240 186–453	0.02
TsF (%) ± SD Confidence interval	32 ± 7 28–36	31 ± 12 18–32	0.5

Responders: Hb ≥11 g/dl and epoetin beta dose <300 IU/kg/week
Non-responders: Hb < 11 g/dl and epoetin dose ≥300 IU/kg/week

Table 5-8: Resistance to epoetin beta treatment in comparison with responders

Figure 5-9 reviews the relationship between haemoglobin and epoetin dose at baseline for patients in maintenance phase (n=322). A negative correlation (r) was found between haemoglobin and epoetin dose at baseline (r= -0.13; p= 0.001), reflecting an inverse relationship between achieved haemoglobin concentration and epoetin dose. The same result was found for month 1 to 6 (month 1: r=-013, p=001; month 2: r=-0.17, p<0.001; month 3: r=-0.17, p<0.001; month 4: r=-0.17, p<0.0001; month 5: r=-0.14, p=0.0004; month 6: r=-0.19, p<0.0001).

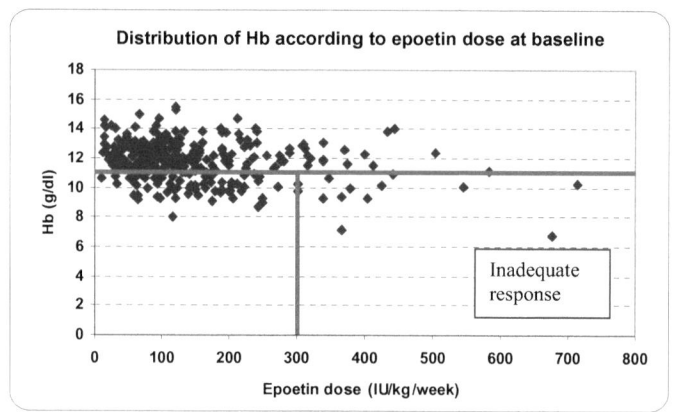

Figure 5-9: Distribution of haemoglobin according to epoetin maintenance dose at baseline

The most common cause for incomplete response to ESAs is iron deficiency. Patients with available transferrin saturation values were classified according to their iron status into three different categories and response to epoetin beta was analysed. The three category groups were as follows: absolute iron deficiency (serum ferritin <100 µg/l), functional iron deficiency (serum ferritin ≥100 µg/l and transferrin saturation <20%) and adequate iron status (serum ferritin levels ≥100 µg/l and transferrin saturation ≥20%). A trend was observed in mean haemoglobin level being lower in patients with absolute and functional iron deficiency compared to patients with adequeate iron status. At baseline and month 4, mean haemoglobin was significantly lower in the category with absolute iron deficiency compared to that with adequate iron status.

Concerning the epoetin dose, patients with functional iron deficiency tended towards higher epoetin dose requirements which were true for patients with absolute iron deficiency only at baseline. Mean epoetin dose of patients with absolute iron deficiency corresponded to the epoetin dose of patients with adequate iron status at month 1-6. Patients with functional iron deficiency required higher epoetin dose at month 3, 4 and 6 compared to the patients with adequate iron stores. More details are given in Table 5-9.

Visits	Group	Number of patients	Mean weekly epoetin dose (IU/kg/week) ± SD	Mean haemoglobin (g/dl) ± SD
Baseline	Adequate iron status	132	144 ± 102	12.2 ± 1.3
	Functional iron deficiency	28	175 ± 97	11.9 ± 1.3
	Absolute iron deficiency	26	190 ± 119**	11.1 ± 1.6+**
Month 1	Adequate iron status	153	133 ± 95	12.1 ± 1.4
	Functional iron deficiency	45	191 ± 99*	11.5 ± 1.5*
	Absolute iron deficiency	17	120 ± 93+	11.7 ± 1.3
Month 2	Adequate iron status	171	140 ± 109	12.1 ± 1.4
	Functional iron deficiency	47	193 ± 120*	11.4 ± 1.5*
	Absolute iron deficiency	24	129 ± 89+	11.8 ± 1.5
Month 3	Adequate iron status	176	144 ± 112	12.0 ± 1.4
	Functional iron deficiency	46	186 ± 108*	11.6 ± 1.6
	Absolute iron deficiency	31	133 ± 105+	11.6 ± 1.4
Month 4	Adequate iron status	169	140 ± 103	12.1 ± 1.2
	Functional iron deficiency	52	184 ± 136*	11.7 ± 1.3
	Absolute iron deficiency	32	141 ± 107	11.5 ± 1.4**
Month 5	Adequate iron status	177	146 ± 113	12.2 ± 1.3
	Functional iron deficiency	47	171 ± 129	11.4 ± 1.3*
	Absolute iron deficiency	33	147 ± 111	11.9 ± 1.6
Month 6	Adequate iron status	171	145 ± 116	12.3 ± 1.3
	Functional iron deficiency	52	186 ± 137*	11.4 ± 1.5*
	Absolute iron deficiency	33	148 ± 127	11.8 ± 1.6

Epoetin dose: *Significant difference observed between patients with adequate iron status and patients with functional iron deficiency at month 1 ($p<0.0001$), month 2 ($p=0.0008$), month 3 ($p=0.0016$), month 4 ($p=0.03$), month 6 ($p=0.01$)
+Significant difference observed between patients with absolute iron deficiency and patients with functional iron deficiency at month 1 ($p<0.003$), month 2 ($p=0.01$), month 3 ($p=0.01$)
**Significant difference observed between patients with absolute iron deficiency and patients with adequate iron status at month 1 ($p=0.04$)
Haemoglobin: *Significant difference observed between patients with adequate iron status and patients with functional iron deficiency at month 1 ($p=0.002$), month 2 ($p=0.0037$), month 5 ($p=0.0008$), month 6 ($p=0.0002$)
+Significant difference observed between patients with absolute iron deficiency and patients with functional iron deficiency at baseline ($p=0.03$)
**Significant difference observed between patients with absolute iron deficiency and patients with adequate iron status at baseline ($p=0.0007$), month 4 ($p=0.03$)
Significance was tested by Kruskal-Wallis method

Table 5-9: Epoetin dose and haemoglobin level in respect of the iron status

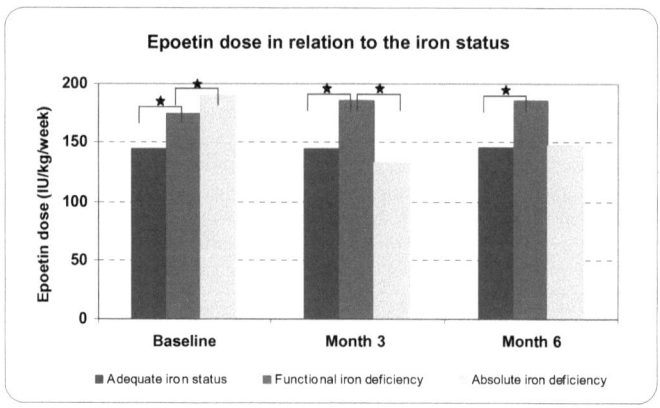

* significant difference

Figure 5-10: Epoetin dose by adequacy of iron status

5.5 Discussion

The survey showed that anaemia was well controlled in the majority of the dialysis patients in Switzerland. Haemoglobin level was in approximately 80% of the patients above the recommended target of 11 g/dl and in 40% above 12 g/dl. Physicians' target haemoglobin was in the majority of the dialysis centres higher than postulated in the recommendations of the EBPG. Physicians' own target haemoglobin level was achieved in approximately half of the patients. Serum ferritin was regularly measured and was in 97% of the patients above the recommended minimum target level of the EBPG. In contrast, in many centres transferrin saturation was not routinely measured. Administered epoetin dose figured in the upper range of the recommendations. Discrepancies were observed concerning administration and dosing frequency of epoetin between the guidelines and the clinical practice in Swiss dialysis centres.

European Best Practice Guidelines recommend target haemoglobin levels of ≥11 g/dl for 85% or more patients and revised EBPG propose a target of ≥11 g/dl in general. Overall, mean haemoglobin was 11.8 g/dl with a median value of 11.9 g/dl. In Swiss dialysis centres, a high quality of anaemia control was achieved, which was higher than the recommended target haemoglobin of the EBPG. 80% of haemodialysis and peritoneal dialysis patients achieved haemoglobin levels of ≥11 g/dl and more than 40% achieved haemoglobin levels of ≥12 g/dl. Even though a high haemoglobin level was obtained in most dialysis patients, 20% of the patients did not reach the recommended target haemoglobin level. Frequent concomitant effects, such as infections and inflammations might have influenced the haemoglobin levels. Haemoglobin levels are expected to be lower in haemodialysis patients than in peritoneal dialysis patients, which is mainly explainable by additional blood loss during haemodialysis, bio-incompatible dialysis membranes, inadequate amount of dialysis and other potential factors. In this survey, haemoglobin was well controlled in both haemodialysis and peritoneal dialysis patients with no difference in achieved haemoglobin levels.

A survey was conducted in all participating centres asking for their centre-specific haemoglobin targets. Physicians' target haemoglobin was in all dialysis centres higher than 11 g/dl. 60% of the participating dialysis centres aimed at partial normalization (Hb ≥12 g/dl) and 23% of the centres at full normalization (Hb ≥13 g/dl) of haemoglobin in their dialysis patients. Target haemoglobin concentrations of Swiss dialysis centres were generally higher than formulated in the recommendations of the EBPG. As a consequence, the proportion of patients achieving physicians' target was lower, especially in dialysis centres where higher targets were aimed at. Physicians' target haemoglobin was achieved in only half of all dialysis patients compared to 85% achieving ≥ 11 g/dl as recommended by the EBPG.

Higher physicians' target haemoglobin level compared to the EBPG can be explained by the fact that different publications demonstrated a beneficial effect at higher haemoglobin targets. Several studies have shown an association between the mortality on dialysis and haemoglobin. The mortality and hospitalization rate decreased at increased haematocrit levels [12, 98]. These findings and the ongoing discussion about the optimal target haemoglobin level might have influenced physicians' target towards higher haemoglobin levels in dialysis patients compared to the EBPG recommendations, even though a recently published study showed a higher incidence of mortality in the higher haematocrit group [115]. Anaemia management in Switzerland was in adherence to the recommendations of the guidelines in most parts and improved over the last half decade towards higher haemoglobin levels compared to the haemoglobin levels (11.7 g/dl in ESAM) achieved in earlier findings [119]. Optimal target haemoglobin still remains to be defined and differences in target haemoglobin between the participating centres reflect this ongoing discussion about the optimal target in dialysis patients.

In order to achieve target haemoglobin levels, chronic renal failure patients must be iron-replete because of the synergistic effect between iron and epoetin. For patients on dialysis, serum ferritin levels between 200-500 µg/l are recommended by the EBPG in order to achieve target haemoglobin concentration. About 90% of the dialysis patients included in "AIMS" had adequate serum ferritin levels (serum ferritin >100 µg/l) and were in 80% of the patients above 200 µg/l. Serum ferritin was regularly and well controlled in all patients included. Physicians tend to observe more carefully the lower limit for serum ferritin in order to ensure optimal haemoglobin level. One third of all centres observed primarily minimal serum ferritin targets without restricting upper limits. This might be due to the fact that most iron stores of dialysis patients, especially of haemodialysis patients, were reduced, as a result of increased blood loss from dialysis, laboratory tests and epoetin administration, which increases the demand for iron [139, 140]. Transferrin saturation was measured in 70% of the patients and was not a routinely performed laboratory parameter in more than one third of all participating dialysis centres. 80% of the patients with measured transferrin saturation achieved adequate (≥ 20%) and 42% optimal (≥ 30%) transferrin saturation targets. Target levels for transferrin saturation corresponded to the minimum targets of the guidelines (>20%) and few centres aimed at the optimal target of 30%. Iron management was not fully in adherence to the EBPG, since serum ferritin targets varied strongly between the dialysis centres and transferrin saturation was not a routinely performed laboratory analysis. It might be advisable to further encourage the implementation of the recommended iron targets of the guidelines in order to optimize iron management and anaemia treatment in dialysis patients.

An adequate iron supply, however, is essential for optimum red cell production and for treatment response with ESAs. Therefore it was expected that iron deficiency would be associated with higher epoetin dose requirements and was analysed for patients with adequate iron stores, functional iron deficiency and for patients with absolute iron deficiency. Epoetin dose was significantly higher in patients with absolute and patients with functional iron deficiency at baseline compared to those with adequate iron stores. Patients with functional iron deficiency tended to require higher epoetin doses than patients with adequate iron status, resulting in lower haemoglobin concentrations. Unexpectedly, patients with iron deficiency did not require higher epoetin doses compared to patients with adequate iron status for month 1 to 6. One explanation might be that patients with absolute iron deficiency have in fact depleted iron stores; however, administered iron may be enough in order to stimulate erythropoiesis adequately. Optimal iron management is nevertheless essential in order to achieve adequate response to ESAs and may also result in a considerable dose reduction and cost-savings.

Administered mean epoetin dose was 149 IU/kg/week (median 122 IU/kg/week) and was in the upper range of the recommended target of 50-150 IU/kg/week of the current guidelines. This elevated epoetin beta dose can be explained by the higher achieved mean haemoglobin concentration, which was above the recommended haemoglobin target of the current guidelines. More than 90% responded to epoetin treatment with epoetin doses of less than 300 IU/kg/week. Epoetin-naïve patients required 20% higher epoetin doses than epoetin-stable patients and achieved target haemoglobin concentrations of 11 g/dl within the recommended 3 months.

The route of administration of erythropoiesis-stimulating agents depends on the patient group and the type of ESA. For haemodialysis patients, the intravenous route may be preferable for reasons of convenience, but the subcutaneous route allows to substantially reduce the dose requirements of epoetin beta. Two third of the patients received epoetin beta by the subcutaneous route of administration and did not significantly change during the observation. Upcoming safety concerns led to the contraindication of the subcutaneous administration of epoetin alfa in 2002. A shift from the predominant subcutaneous to the intravenous administration was also expected for epoetin beta; however, this was not confirmed by the findings of the survey. In contrast to the recommendation, 90% of the patients received epoetin beta as a 1x weekly dosing regimen already at therapy initiation. Approximately two third of the patients with intravenous administration of epoetin received it as a 1x weekly dosing scheme, even though there is lack of evidence to support this dosing regimen in haemodialysis patients. The findings show that there are differences between the recommendations and the clinical practice regarding the dosing regimen of epoetin beta.

In conclusion, target haemoglobin level remains the most controversial issue in the therapy of renal anaemia. On the one hand, complete normalization of haemoglobin concentrations appeared possible in the majority of patients as demonstrated in different phase I and II trials with rHuEPO [141]. On the other hand, concerns arised about the fact that normalization of haemoglobin was associated with adverse outcome, in particular cardiovascular events [142, 143], hypertension [144] and vascular access thrombosis [145]. There is evidence that haemoglobin concentration should be raised above 11 g/dl, but the optimum target haemoglobin level above this concentration remains still unclear. In a large ongoing observational study, higher Hb levels were associated with a decreased risk of mortality and hospitalization [146]. A prospective Canadian study of haemodialysis patients found a 1 g/dl decrease of haemoglobin to be associated with a significant increase in mortality [147]. In contrast, the study of Besarab was interrupted because the mortality rate was higher in the "high" haemoglobin group compared to the "lower" haemoglobin group [115]. In all of these trials, quality of life parameters were significantly improved and some trials indicated survival benefits with increased haemoglobin levels. Higher target haemoglobin will probably have major implications on treatment costs, since higher epoetin dose will be necessary in order to achieve or maintain target haemoglobin levels. On the one hand, higher haemoglobin targets may increase costs of epoetin therapy but on the other hand, potential beneficial effects such as reduced hospitalization rate and reduced heart failure rate have to be counterbalanced against increased treatment costs. So far, there are not sufficient data available to perform pharma-economic calculations of that kind. Therefore, the discussion about the optimal target haemoglobin level and the individualized anaemia therapy in patients with chronic kidney disease is still an ongoing process.

6. Management of anaemia in dialyzed patients in Switzerland: a survey comparing a once a week with a 2-3 times weekly administration of epoetin beta

N. Lötscher[1], D. Teta[2], S. Maack[1], D. Kiss[3], P.-Y. Martin[4], M. Burnier[2]*

1   Roche (Pharma) Switzerland Ltd, P.O. Box, CH-4153 Reinach, Switzerland
2   CHUV, Department of Internal Medicine, Nephrology, P.O. Box, CH-1011 Lausanne, Switzerland
4   Kantonsspital Liestal, Department of Nephrology, P.O. Box, CH-4410 Liestal, Switzerland
5   HCUG, Department of Internal Medicine, Nephrology, P.O. Box, CH-1211 Geneva, Switzerland

*Corresponding author:

Tel.:   +41 21 314 11 54
E-mail: michel.burnier@hospvd.ch

Oral presentation by D. Teta[1] at the SGIM congress
(Schweizerische Gesellschaft für Innere Medizin), Lausanne 2004
The abstract was published in:
Swiss Medical Forum; 4: Supplementum 17: 7

6.1 Abstract

Aim: The purpose of this analysis was to evaluate the quality of the control of anaemia obtained with a 1x weekly or a 2-3x weekly administration of epoetin beta in dialyzed patients in Switzerland. In addition, the survey assessed the clinical practice of anaemia treatment and the potential benefits of the 1x weekly administration of epoetin beta.

Method: 368 dialyzed patients (58% male, 42% female, medium age 63.5 years, mostly pretreated with epoetin) of 28 dialysis centres in Switzerland were included in this practice-based survey. Anaemia treatment with epoetin beta (1x weekly versus more frequent administration) in clinical practice was observed for 12 months. All patients were administered iron supplementation if required.

Result: The analysis was performed in 340 patients (207 patients in the 1x weekly and 133 in the 2-3x weekly group). At baseline, the two groups were comparable in terms of gender, haemoglobin, route of administration, serum ferritin and transferrin saturation. Differences between groups were observed in terms of age and epoetin beta dose at baseline. Baseline serum ferritin was 418 ±304 µg/l in the 1x weekly and 402 ±286 µg/l in the 2-3x weekly group and remained above 300 µg/l throughout the observation period in both groups. Mean haemoglobin levels at baseline, after 1, 3 and 6 months were 11.9 ± 1.4, 11.8 ± 1.3, 11.8 ± 1.2 and 11.9 ± 1.3 g/dl in the 1x weekly group, and 11.5 ± 1.5, 11.7 ± 1.4, 11.8 ± 1.6 and 11.7 ± 1.6 g/dl in the 2-3x weekly group. No statistical significance was found between the two groups. Mean epoetin beta dosages at baseline, after 1, 3 and 6 months were 121 ± 94, 120 ± 94, 130 ± 118 and 129 ± 114 IU/kg/week in the 1x weekly group and 178 ± 119, 178 ± 114, 184 ± 116, and 197 ± 131 IU/kg/week in the 2-3x weekly group. The mean weekly epoetin beta dosage was significantly lower in the 1x weekly group than in the 2-3x weekly group ($p<0.05$). This difference occurred already at baseline and remained throughout the observation period. Both regimens were well tolerated. 38% of the treating physicians considered the reduced number of injections and 33% the reduced time spent in hospital as the main advantages of the 1x weekly administration of epoetin beta.

Conclusions: These data show that anaemia of a large proportion of dialyzed patients can be effectively managed with a 1x weekly administration of epoetin beta. The 1x weekly regimen appears to be as effective in maintaining the haemoglobin level as a 2-3x weekly dosing regimen. The 1x weekly regimen results in a reduced workload for the medical staff, a higher patient convenience and a better patient compliance.

Key words: Anaemia, anaemia management, epoetin, epoetin beta, once weekly, dosing frequency, end-stage renal disease, dialysis

6.2 Introduction

The survey *AnaemIa Management in dialysis patients in Switzerland* "AIMS" was designed as a prospective, 12 months practice-based, open-intervention survey and was performed from June 2002 until December 2004. Data regarding anaemia management, causes and co- morbidities of chronic kidney disease of the patients included in "AIMS" were collected. Earlier, we analysed anaemia management in Swiss dialysis centres and compared the results with the European Best Practice Guidelines (EBPG) for the management of anaemia in patients with chronic renal failure. Results of these two analyses demonstrated that anaemia was well controlled in dialysis patients cared in Swiss dialysis centres and that the majority of the patients achieved target haemoglobin recommended by the guidelines. In this third analysis, we assessed the relevance and the efficacy of the 1x weekly subcutaneous administration of epoetin beta in dialysis patients in Switzerland.

Subcutaneous administration allows to reduce epoetin dose as well as the dosing frequency. Numerous clinical studies have demonstrated that the subcutaneous administration of epoetin is more efficacious than the intravenous route, allowing the maintenance of the same target haemoglobin levels at lower epoetin doses [15, 40, 82]. Beside the cost-effectivity of the subcutaneous administration of epoetin beta, pharmacokinetic evaluation of subcutaneous administration in healthy persons showed a prolonged elimination half-time compared to intravenous administration. This pharmacokinetic advantage of the subcutaneous administration allowed to reduce the dosing intervals of epoetin beta from 2-3x weekly to 1x weekly administration in stable chronic kidney disease patients. In continuous ambulatory peritoneal dialysis patients and in pre-dialysis patients 1x weekly administration of epoetin beta proved to be as effective and safe in maintaining a stable haemoglobin level as the 3x weekly dosing regimen [79].

In stable haemodialysis patients, two large, randomized, controlled trials were conducted proving the same efficacy of 1x weekly subcutaneous administration as the 2-3x weekly administration of the same total weekly epoetin dose [77, 78]. The study of Weiss et al. demonstrated that 1x weekly administration of epoetin beta was effective in maintaining haemoglobin levels in stable haemodialysis patients without significant dose increase and the study of Locatelli et al. showed therapeutic equivalence between the 1x weekly and the more frequent administration of epoetin beta [77, 78]. These data led to the approval of the 1x weekly dosing regimen of epoetin beta in stable patients with renal anaemia in September 2001.

In clinical practice, epoetin has been administered 2-3x weekly for more than 10 years. Clinical studies have proven efficacy of the 1x weekly subcutaneous administration of epoetin beta in stable haemodialysis patients, but there was still limited experience regarding the 1x weekly regimen since the European approval in 2001. The aim of this survey was to assess the relevance of the 1x weekly dosing regimen of epoetin beta in clinical practice in Switzerland and to investigate the efficacy and safety of the 1x weekly dosing regimen compared to the 2-3x weekly administration. Benefits of the 1x weekly subcutaneous dosing regimen are associated with reduced dosing frequency, reduced workload for medical staff and increased patient compliance with self-administration. The second objective of the survey concerned the question to know whether the prolonged dosing interval of epoetin beta was feasible and beneficial in dialyzed patients in Switzerland.

6.3 Subjects and methods

Patients and data collection

The survey was conducted as a prospective, open-intervention and practice-based survey. 28 Swiss dialysis centres participated and 368 patients were registered, 340 patients thereof were eligible. The aim of the survey was to assess the relevance and the efficacy of the 1x weekly dosing regimen in Swiss dialysis centres. At patient registration, aetiology of chronic renal failure, concomitant disease, dialysis treatment, laboratory parameters (haemoglobin, serum ferritin, and transferrin saturation), dry weight, pre-treatment with epoetin and current epoetin treatment (dose, route of administration and frequency) were registered. During the observation period of 12 months, efficacy parameters (haemoglobin and epoetin dose), route of administration and dosing frequency of epoetin beta were requested to be documented monthly on a pre-printed clinical report form.

Inclusion and exclusion criteria were evaluated at survey entry. The inclusion criteria were the following: Patients ≥ 18 years old either on haemodialysis or peritoneal dialysis; patients pre-treated with epoetin or epoetin-naïve patients with renal anaemia. The exclusion criteria were defined as follows: Patients with iron deficiency (< 200 µg/l), deficiency of vitamin B_{12} (<200 ng/l) and/or folic acid (2 µg/l), patients with unstable angina pectoris, untreated hypertension, haemoglobinopathy and/or haemolysis. Pregnant or nursing patients were not allowed for survey inclusion. Dialysis centres documented anaemia treatment with epoetin beta according to their clinical practice. Dosing schedule of epoetin beta was recommended according to the EBPG and/or the prescribing information.

Prescribing information of epoetin beta: Correction phase: The recommended dosage for subcutaneous administration is 3x 20 IU/kg/week and for intravenous administration 3x 40 IU/kg/week. Dosage may be doubled after four weeks if haematocrit increase was smaller than 0.5% per week. Further dose increments of 3x 20 IU/kg/week are allowed if necessary. Maintenance phase: 50% dose reduction of the last administered epoetin beta dose. In case of subcutaneous administration, the weekly dose can be given as an injection once a week and stable patients on a 1x weekly regimen can be switched to once every two weeks administration. The maximum dose should not exceed 720 IU/kg/week [75, 81].

European Best Practice Guidelines (EBPG): Initial epoetin administration: The starting dose of epoetin should be between 50-150 IU/kg/week (4,000-8,000 IU/week), administered 2-3x a week. For intravenous administration, the starting dose should be in the upper range (typically 6,000 IU/week) three times a week. If the increase of haemoglobin concentration was <1.0 g/dl over a 4 week period, the dose of epoetin should be increased by 25%. If the increase of Hb level was > 2.5 g/dl or exceeded the target Hb concentration, the weekly dose of epoetin should be reduced by 25-50%. Recommended target haemoglobin level is ≥ 11 g/dl in chronic renal failure patients [40, 82].

All patients included in the survey should be iron-repleted. For patients on dialysis, optimal serum ferritin levels between 200-500 µg/l and transferrin saturation of 30-40% are recommended. Iron supplementation should be followed according to the EBPG [40, 82]. All medications and treatments for renal anaemia and other concomitant diseases were permitted.

The received filled-in data report forms were examined in respect of completeness of mandatory data and validated prior data entry. Patients who did not fulfill the inclusion or exclusion criteria were excluded. All patients who received at least one dose of epoetin beta were included in the analysis. Last observation carried forward method (LOCF) was used for value replacement. Subgroup analyses were performed comparing the 1x weekly with the 2-3x weekly administration of epoetin beta. The primary efficacy parameters of the subgroup analysis were area under the curve (AUC) for haemoglobin and for mean weekly epoetin beta dose per kilogram bodyweight. Secondary outcome parameters were mean haemoglobin concentration and mean weekly epoetin dose per kilogram body weight, as well as changes in haemoglobin from baseline. Safety parameters were adverse events occurring during the survey.

Statistics

All statistical tests were performed using SAS, version 8.1 (SAS Institute, Cary, NC, USA), Excel 2002 or Epi-Info®, version 3.2. A sample size of 146 (72.4 patients per group) was computed in order to achieve a 95% power to detect a difference in mean haemoglobin of 0.6 g/dl between the two groups with a known standard deviation of 1.0 g/dl and a significance level (alpha) of 0.05 (confidence interval of 95%) using a two-sided two-sample t-test. Assuming a drop-out rate of 20%, a total of 90 patients per group have to be enrolled. AUC for haemoglobin and mean weekly epoetin beta dose were calculated using a covariance model. Confidence intervals were used to compare haemoglobin concentrations of the two treatment groups and an equivalence range of ± 0.6 g/dl was chosen to detect differences in mean AUC for haemoglobin between the two treatment groups. A two-sample t-test on a 95% confidence level was used to compare differences in epoetin beta dose.

Kaplan-Meier was used for mortality analysis over time. Mortality was assessed in respect of different haemoglobin levels (Hb ≥11 g/dl vs Hb < 11 g/dl; Hb ≥12 g/dl vs Hb <12 g/dl). Descriptive statistics were used to analyse anaemia treatment in Swiss dialysis centres including 95% confidence interval, mean, median and standard deviation for the primary variables (haemoglobin and epoetin beta dose). Categorical variables were compared using the χ^2-test and continuous variables using Students' t-test, Wilcoxon two-sample and Kruskal-Wallis test, where appropriate. All statistical tests were two-sided and the significance was tested on a 0.05 p-value.

6.4 Results

6.4.1 Patient characteristics

Six months data of "AIMS" are presented in this article. 368 patients from 28 Swiss dialysis centres were included in this survey, 340 thereof were eligible. 95% were on haemodialysis and 5% on peritoneal dialysis. Mean age of the studied population was 63.5 years, ranging from 18 to 91. 58% of the population were male and 42% were female. 18 of 340 patients were epoetin-naïve patients.

207 patients received epoetin beta as a 1x weekly and 133 as a 2-3x weekly treatment regimen. 6% of the 1x weekly group (n= 14) and 3% of the 2-3x weekly group (n=4) were epoetin-naïve patients without significant difference between the two groups (p=0.131, χ^2-test).

Variables at baseline	1x weekly (n=207)	2-3x weekly (n=133)
Mean Age (years)	65 ± 14.5*	61 ± 14.5*
Range	18–90	22–91
Male (n)	116	82
Female (n)	91	51
Body weight (kg)	68.6 ± 15.1	70.9 ± 15.5
Range	40–129	40–122
Systolic blood pressure (mmHg)	159 ± 21 (n=83)	166 ± 27 (n=37)
Diastolic blood pressure (mmHg)	84 ± 14 (n=83)	90 ±18 (n=37)
Haemoglobin (g/dl)	11.9 ± 1.4	11.6 ± 1.5
Range	8.0–15.5	6.8–14.7
Mean weekly epoetin beta dose	121.3 ± 93.5**	177.7 ± 119.1**
Median weekly epoetin beta dose	98.4	155.8
Range (IU/kg/week)	12.9–714.3	11.2–676.7
Serum ferritin (µg/l)	418 ± 304	401 ± 308
Transferrin saturation (%)	31 ± 14 (n=105)	30 ± 16 (n=66)

*p=0.02 for age; **p<0.0001 for epoetin dose at baseline

Table 6-1: Baseline patient characteristics of the 1x weekly and the 2-3x weekly group

Patient characteristics for body weight, blood pressure, haemoglobin concentration at baseline, ferritin and transferrin saturation were comparable without significant difference. Mean age was significantly higher in the 1x weekly group (p=0.02, χ^2-test). At baseline, epoetin beta dose was significantly higher in the 2-3x weekly group compared to the 1x weekly group (p< 0.00001, Students' t-test). There were more male than female patients in both treatment groups. Baseline characteristics of both treatment groups are shown in Table 6-1.

Diagnosis	Total		1x weekly (n=207)		2-3x weekly (n=133)		p value*
	n	%	n	%	n	%	
Diabetic nephropathy	71	20.9	47	22.7	24	18.1	0.37
Glomerulonephritis	79	23.2	46	22.2	33	24.8	0.67
PN / IN	58	17.1	37	17.9	21	15.8	0.72
HT / vascular causes	72	21.2	41	19.8	31	23.3	0.53
PKD	27	7.9	15	7.3	12	9.0	0.70
Neoplasm / tumours	9	2.6	6	2.9	3	2.3	0.49[1]
Unclear	13	3.8	8	3.9	5	3.8	0.96
Miscellaneous causes	10	2.9	7	3.4	3	2.3	0.31[1]
Missing	9	2.6	3	1.5	6	4.5	0.75[1]

*p value comparing 1x weekly vs 2-3x weekly
[1]Fisher exact test for values n < 5
No significant difference between groups
PN= pyelonephritis; IN=interstitial nephritis; HT=hypertension; PKD=polycystic kidney disease
Multiple entries possible, therefore not cumulative

Table 6-2: Aetiology of end-stage renal disease in the 1x weekly and 2-3x weekly group

Most frequent concomitant diseases in the 1x weekly and the 2-3x weekly group were coronary artery disease (29.0% and 20.3%, respectively) heart failure (17.3% and 15.0%, respectively), hypertension (58.5% and 63.9%, respectively) and diabetes (30.0% and 23.3%, respectively), with no significant differences between the groups. Cardiac diseases (without hypertension) were reported in 50% of patients in the 1x weekly and in 43% of the 2-3x weekly group. Hyperparathyroidism, hepatological and metabolic disorders occurred more frequently in the 2-3x weekly group. Only few patients with hyperparathyroidism (6 patients), hepatological (7) and metabolic disorders (7) were reported within this survey and the predominance in the 2-3x times weekly group does not seem to be of any relevance. Table 6-3 provides an overview of concomitant diseases in both treatment groups.

Concomitant diseases	Total		1x weekly (n=207)		2-3x weekly (n=133)		p value
	n	%	n	%	n	%	
Coronary artery disease	87	25.5	60	29.0	27	20.3	0.07
Congestive heart failure	56	16.5	36	17.3	20	15.0	0.56
Hypertension	206	60.6	121	58.5	85	63.9	0.32
Other cardiac diseases	18	5.3	8	3.9	10	7.5	0.14
Diabetes[2]	93	27.4	62	30.0	31	23.3	0.18
Vascular diseases	17	5.0	10	4.8	7	5.3	0.85
Metabolic disorders	7	2.0	1	0.5	6	4.5	0.02*[1]
Hyperparathyroidism	6	1.8	1	0.5	5	3.7	0.04*[1]
CsA nephropathy	3	0.9	1	0.5	2	1.5	0.56[1]
COPD	6	1.8	3	1.4	3	2.3	0.68[1]
Hepatological disorders	7	2.0	1	0.5	6	4.5	0.02*[1]
Cancer (CA)	7	2.0	3	1.4	4	3.0	0.44[1]
Bone diseases	4	1.2	2	1.0	2	1.5	0.65[1]
Other diseases	7	2.0	3	1.4	4	3.0	0.44[1]

*p= significant
[1] Fisher exact test for values < 5
[2] Diabetes overall (n=93): reported as concomitant disease (n=79), 53 thereof in the 1x weekly and 26 in the 2-3x weekly group (p=0.2); reported as primary diagnosis (n=71)
Multiple entries possible, therefore not cumulative

Table 6-3: Concomitant diseases of the 1x weekly and the 2-3x weekly group

6.4.2 Efficacy of the 1x weekly dosing scheme of epoetin beta

Efficacy of 1x weekly vs 2-3x weekly administration of epoetin beta

Mean haemoglobin remained stable in both groups and no significant changes occurred between baseline and month 6 within the groups. A comparison of mean haemoglobin between the groups is depicted in Figure 6-1. For the 1x weekly group, mean haemoglobin levels were 11.9 ± 1.4 g/dl (95% CI: 11.7–12.1 g/dl) at baseline, 11.8 ± 1.3 g/dl (95% CI: 11.5–12.0 g/dl) at month 1, 11.7 ± 1.3 g/dl (95% CI: 11.5–11.9 g/dl) at month 2, 11.8 ± 1.2 g/dl (95% CI: 11.5–11.9 g/dl) at month 3, 11.9 ± 1.1 g/dl (95% CI: 11.7–12.0 g/dl) at month 4, 11.9 ± 1.3 g/dl (95% CI: 11.6–12.0 g/dl) at month 5 and 11.9 ± 1.3 g/dl (95% CI: 11.7–12.1 g/dl) at month 6. For the 2-3x weekly group, mean haemoglobin levels were 11.5 ± 1.5 g/dl (95% CI: 11.2–11.8 g/dl) at baseline, 11.7 ± 1.4 g/dl (95% CI: 11.4–11.9 g/dl) at month 1, 11.7 ± 1.6 g/dl (95% CI: 11.4–12.0 g/dl) at month 2, 11.8 ± 1.6 g/dl (95% CI: 11.4–12.1 g/dl) at month 3, 11.8 ± 1.4 g/dl (95% CI: 11.5–12.1 g/dl) at month 4, 11.8 ± 1.5 g/dl (95% CI: 11.4–12.1 g/dl) at month 5, 11.7 ± 1.6 g/dl (95% CI: 11.4–12.0 g/dl) at month 6.

The difference in least squares mean AUC for haemoglobin between the two groups (16.81) and the 95% confidence interval of this value (CI:-14.67–48.29) were within the pre-specified reference range of $\pm$ 90 (0.5 g/dl for 180 days). No significant difference in haemoglobin level occurred between both treatment groups (p=0.38) for all six months.

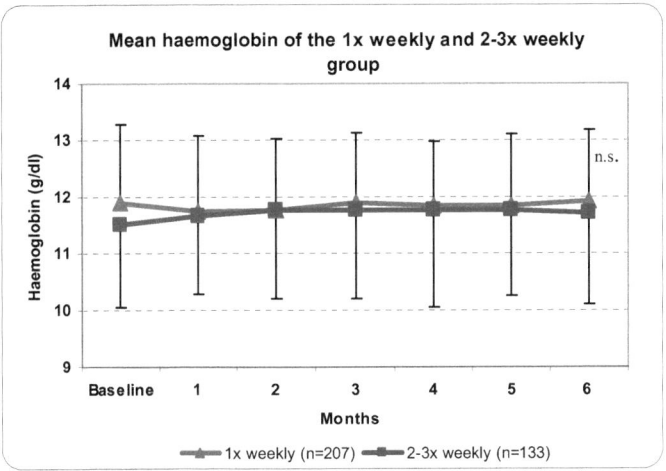

n.s.=not significant difference between both groups for all six months

Figure 6-1: Mean haemoglobin over time in the two treatment groups

Mean weekly epoetin beta dosage was significantly lower in the 1x weekly group than in the 2-3x weekly group (p<0.0001). The difference in mean epoetin beta dose was at baseline apparent and remained throughout the whole observation period of six months. Within the groups (1x weekly and 2-3x weekly group), no significant difference occurred for epoetin beta dose between baseline and month 6 (p>0.05). Figure 6-2 and Table 6-4 provide more detailed efficacy results of both treatment groups.

Mean epoetin beta dose and confidence intervals were as follows: In the 1x weekly group, mean epoetin beta dose was 121 ± 94 IU/kg/week (95% CI: 105–138 IU/kg/week) at baseline, 120 ± 94 IU/kg/week (95% CI: 103–137 IU/kg/week) at month 1, 127 ± 109 IU/kg/week (95% CI: 107–147 IU/kg/week) at month 2, 130 ± 118 IU/kg/week (95% CI: 109–152 IU/kg/week) at month 3, 130 ± 117 IU/kg/week (95% CI: 109–151 IU/kg/week) at month 4, 132 ±121 IU/kg/week (95% CI: 110–153 IU/kg/week) at month 5 and 129 ± 114 IU/kg/week (95% CI: 108–149 IU/kg/week) at month 6. In the 2-3x weekly group, mean epoetin beta dosage was 178 ± 119 IU/kg/week (95% CI: 151–205 IU/kg/week) at baseline, 178 ± 114 IU/kg/week (95% CI: 152–204 IU/kg/week) at month 1, 188 ± 120 IU/kg/week (95% CI: 161–215 IU/kg/week) at month 2, 184 ± 116 IU/kg/week (95% CI: 158–210 IU/kg/week) at month 3, 188 ± 134 IU/kg/week (95% CI: 158–218 IU/kg/week) at month 4, 185 ± 123 IU/kg/week (95% CI: 157–212 IU/kg/week) at month 5 and 197 ± 131 IU/kg/week (95% CI: 167–227 IU/kg/week) at month 6. Median weekly epoetin beta dose at baseline and month 6 was 98 and 101 IU/kg/week in the 1x weekly and 156 and 164 IU/kg in the 2-3x weekly group, respectively.

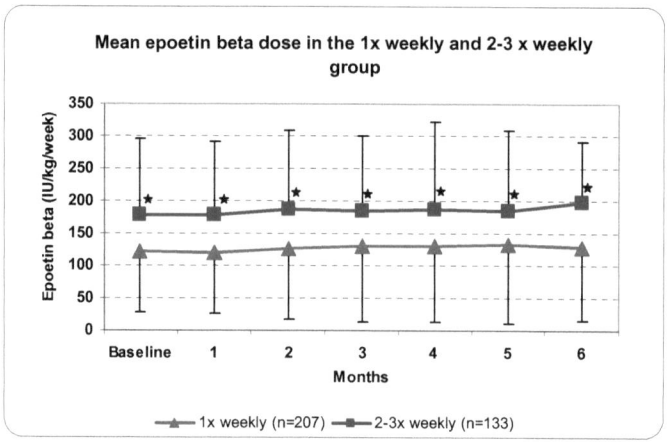

* significant difference between the 1x weekly and the 2-3x weekly group for all six months (p< 0.05)

Figure 6-2: Mean epoetin beta doses for the 1x weekly and the 2-3 x weekly treatment group

We also analysed mean weekly epoetin beta dose of stable dialysis patients in maintenance phase (n=322). At baseline and after month 6, mean weekly epoetin beta dose of stable dialysis patients in the 1x weekly group (n=193 patients) was 121 ± 94 IU/kg/week (median: 100 IU/kg/week) and 125 ± 104 IU/kg/week (median: 97.2 IU/kg/week), respectively. In the 2-3x weekly group (n=129), mean epoetin beta dose of the stable patients was 177 ± 119 IU/kg/week at baseline (median: 149.3 IU/kg/week) and 198 ± 131 IU/kg/week (median: 163.9 IU/kg/week) at month 6. Epoetin beta dose increased by 11.8% in the 2-3x weekly group without significant difference (p=0.18, Students' t-test)., Mean epoetin beta dose of the stable dialysis patients remained stable over six months in the 1x weekly group and was significantly lower compared to the 2-3x weekly group (p<0.0001).

At baseline, mean serum ferritin values were comparable between the 1x weekly and the 2-3x weekly group. For months 1 to 6, mean serum ferritin levels were significantly lower in the 2-3x weekly group (see Table 6-5). However, mean serum ferritin remained above 360 µg/l in both treatment groups throughout the observation period and was above the threshold of 200 µg/l recommended by the EBPG. In the 1x weekly group, mean serum ferritin values were 418 ± 304 µg/l at baseline and 462 ± 301 µg/l at month 6. In the 2-3x weekly group mean serum ferritin values were 402 ± 286 µg/l at baseline and 377 ± 329 µg/l at month 6. Mean serum ferritin values are provided in Table 6-5. A difference in mean serum ferritin values was also observed for stable patients between both groups at month 1 to 6 (data not shown). Transferrin saturation was not regularly measured in all participating centres. Values were available for 245 patients. No significant difference occurred between the two groups. In the 1x weekly group, mean transferrin saturation was 31 ± 14% at baseline, 34 ± 17% at month 1, 31 ± 15% at month 2, 29 ± 13% at month 3, 30 ± 15% at month 4, 29 ± 13% at month 5 and 29 ± 15% at month 6. In the 2-3x weekly group, mean transferrin saturation was 30 ± 16% at baseline, 33 ± 18% at month 1, 33 ± 15% at month 2, 25 ± 11% at month 3, 28 ± 15% at month 4, 28 ± 15 at month 5 and 27 ± 11% at month 6.

Table 6-4 and Table 6-5 provide a summary of efficacy parameters and serum ferritin levels for both groups.

Haemoglobin	g/dl	Baseline	Month 1	Month 2	Month 3	Month 4	Month 5	Month 6
1x weekly*	Mean	11.9	11.8	11.7	11.8	11.9	11.9	11.9
(n=207)	SD	1.4	1.3	1.3	1.2	1.1	1.3	1.3
2-3x weekly*	Mean	11.5	11.7	11.7	11.8	11.8	11.8	11.7
(n=133)	SD	1.5	1.4	1.6	1.6	1.4	1.5	1.6
Difference	g/dl	0.4	0.1	0.03	0	0.1	0.1	0.2

*1x weekly group vs 2-3x weekly group, baseline and month 1-6, statistically not significant

Epoetin dose	IU/kg/week	Baseline	Month 1	Month 2	Month 3	Month 4	Month 5	Month 6
1x weekly	Mean	121	120	127	130	130	132	129
(n=207)	SD	94	94	109	118	117	121	114
2-3x weekly	Mean	178	178	188	184	188	185	197
(n=133)	SD	119	114	120	116	134	123	131
Difference	%	46.5	47.6	47.8	41.6	44.8	40.2	53.2

*1x weekly group vs 2-3x weekly group, month 1-6, statistically significant (p<0.0001)

Table 6-4: Mean epoetin beta dose and haemoglobin level at baseline and month 1 to 6

Serum ferritin	µg/l	Baseline	Month 1	Month 2	Month 3	Month 4	Month 5	Month 6
1x weekly*	Mean	418	407	504	478	471	460	462
(n=207)	SD	304	194	316	332	333	328	301
2-3x weekly*	Mean	402	445	434	392	364	375	377
(n=133)	SD	286	297	341	339	323	344	329
P value (t-test)		0.20	0.0004	<0.0001	0.0004	<0.0001	0.0003	0.0002

*Mean serum ferritin was significantly different between the groups (p=0.0002; Students' t-test)

Table 6-5: Mean serum ferritin at baseline and month 1 to 6

Efficacy of the 1x weekly dose of epoetin beta according to the route of administration

The efficacy of the subcutaneous administration was analysed in respect of the administration frequency. 1x weekly s.c. administration was compared with the 2-3x weekly s.c. administration of epoetin beta. At baseline, 152 patients received epoetin beta 1x weekly s.c. and 89 patients as a 2-3x weekly s.c. administration. Mean haemoglobin level was significantly lower in the 2-3x weekly group at baseline (p=0.02; Students' t-test), and was comparable with no significant difference in both treatment groups for month 1-6 (p>0.5; Students't-test). Mean epoetin dose was significantly lower in the 1x weekly s.c. compared to the 2-3x weekly s.c. group, as illustrated in Table 6-6 (p<0.05; Students't-test).

In the next analysis, we compared the efficacy of the intravenous route of administration in respect of administration frequency (1x weekly i.v. vs 2-3x weekly i.v.). At baseline, 99 patients received epoetin beta intravenously, 55 thereof received it as a 1x weekly dosing regimen. Baseline haemoglobin levels were comparable between both groups. Haemoglobin concentration of the 2-3x weekly i.v. group was reduced from 11.6 at baseline to 11.0 g/dl at month 3, whereas mean epoetin requirement increased by more than 25% (205 IU/kg/week at month 4). Epoetin dose requirement was elevated in the 2-3x weekly i.v. group compared to the 1x weekly i.v. group. More details are given in Table 6-7.

Parameters	Group (s.c.)	Baseline	Month 1	Month 2	Month 3	Month 4	Month 5	Month 6
Number of patients	1x weekly	152	147	144	144	152	152	152
	2-3x weekly	89	94	91	90	85	84	84
Mean haemo-globin (g/dl)	1x weekly	12.0	11.8	11.9	11.9	11.9	11.9	12.0
	2-3x weekly	11.5	11.8	12.0	12.1	12.1	12.1	12.0
P value Hb		0.02	0.63	0.71	0.24	0.29	0.46	0.79
Mean epoetin dose*	1x weekly	127	124	124	123	136	138	134
	2-3x weekly	186	182	193	184	178	180	197
P value Epo		<0.001	<0.001	<0.001	<0.001	0.02	0.02	0.001
Mean serum ferritin (µg/l)	1x weekly	383	400	469	438	462	448	452
	2-3x weekly	421	442	417	389	356	378	391

*IU/kg/week

Table 6-6: Comparison of 1x weekly s.c. versus 2-3x weekly s.c. administration

Parameters	Group (i.v.)	Baseline	Month 1	Month 2	Month 3	Month 4	Month 5	Month 6
Number of patients	1x weekly	55	60	63	63	55	55	55
	2-3x weekly	44	39	42	43	48	49	49
Mean haemo-globin (g/dl)	1x weekly	11.8	11.7	11.3	11.4	11.8	11.7	11.7
	2-3x weekly	11.6	11.3	11.1	11.0	11.3	11.3	11.3
Mean epoetin dose*	1x weekly	107	113	134	146	112	113	113
	2-3x weekly	161	168	177	185	205	192	198
Mean serum ferritin (µg/l)	1x weekly	516	423	586	569	496	495	492
	2-3x weekly	363	451	471	399	379	370	353

No p value was computed, since patient groups did not fulfill the minimum sample size criteria
*(IU/kg/week)

Table 6-7: Comparison of 1x weekly i.v. versus 2-3x weekly i.v. administration

Benefits of the 1x weekly administration of epoetin beta

Epoetin dose requirements were significantly higher in the 2-3x weekly group independently of the route of administration. Higher mean weekly epoetin beta dose was more likely to be given as 2-3x weekly administration and lower epoetin dose as a 1x weekly dosing regimen, which was prooven in a univariate analysis (p<0.0001).

61% of all patients included in this survey received epoetin beta as a 1x weekly treatment regimen. 38% of the treating physicians considered the reduced number of injections and 33% the reduced in-hospital time as the main advantages of the 1x weekly administration of epoetin beta. 9% of the physicians stated to continue with the 2-3x weekly administration of epoetin.

6.4.3 Safety parameters

41 of 340 patients interrupted the survey before survey end and their data reports were not completed for all six months but were at least available for baseline. 21 of 41 patients with early interruption of the survey were lost to follow up due to transfer to other dialy-

sis centres (n=7 patients), study medication interruptions/changes (n= 4 patients) or other/unknown reasons (n=10 patients), 7 patients were transplanted and 13 patients died within the 6 months observation period. Death of patients was not associated with the administration of epoetin beta, since no drug-related adverse events were reported to Swissmedic or to the manufacturer.

In the 1x weekly group, 11 patients died, 4 patients were transplanted and 14 were lost to follow-up. In the 2-3x weekly group, 2 patients died, 3 patients were transplanted and 7 were lost to follow up. No significant difference was detected between both groups in respect of mortality and drop-outs (p>0.05; χ^2-test). The overall mortality rate for dialysis patients was 3.8% in 6 months, the registered overall survival rate 96.2% (see Figure 6-3).

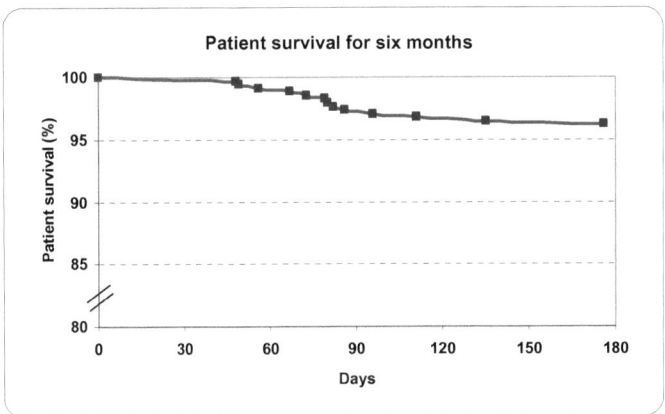

Figure 6-3: Survival curve of dialysis patients for six months

The mortality rate of dialysis patients was observed at different thresholds of mean haemoglobin concentrations. Mean survival rate was similar for patients with haemoglobin ≥11 g/dl (7 patients died; 4.8%) compared to haemoglobin <11 g/dl (6 patients died; 3.1%), as illustrated in Figure 6-4. At a threshold of 12 g/dl, 3.4% (n=10 of 293 patients) in the lower haemoglobin group and 6.4% (n=3 of 47 patients) of the patients in the higher haemoglobin group deceased, with no differences noted between the groups.

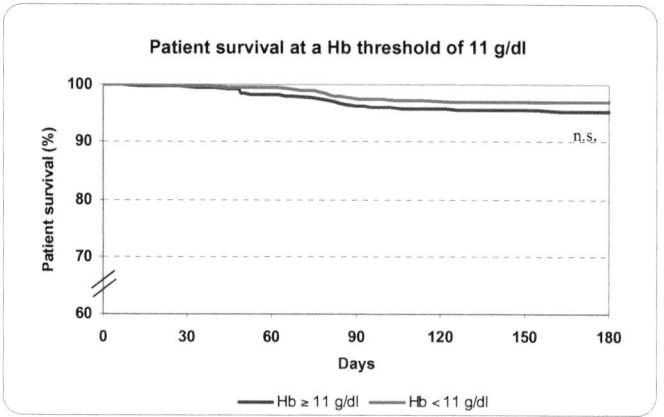

n.s.=no significant difference between both groups

Figure 6-4: Patient survival noted at different haemoglobin thresholds

6.5 Discussion

The findings demonstrate that epoetin beta was in about 60% of all dialysis patients administered as a 1x weekly dosing regimen with comparable efficacy to the 2-3x weekly administration of epoetin beta. Mean weekly epoetin beta dose was significantly lower in the 1x weekly group compared to the 2-3x weekly group. This difference was already apparent at baseline. Beside the difference in baseline epoetin beta dose, the groups were well balanced in terms of diagnosis, concomitant diseases, haemoglobin, and baseline serum ferritin and transferrin saturation. Baseline serum ferritin remained above 360 µg/l in both groups, fulfilling the required optimal target by the EBPG for serum ferritin [40, 82]. The 1x weekly dosing regimen of epoetin beta showed to be effective and to have a safety profile similar to the one of the 2-3x weekly dosing regimen. Higher weekly epoetin beta doses were more likely to be given as 2-3x weekly administration and lower weekly epoetin doses as a 1x weekly dosing regimen.

For more than 10 years, epoetin had been administered as a 2-3x weekly dosing regimen and clinical experience of the 1x weekly administration was limited, since it was only in 2001 that the 1x weekly subcutaneous dosing regimen of epoetin beta was approved for patients with renal anaemia by the EMEA, who were stable on a 2-3x weekly administration of epoetin beta. Nevertheless, the findings indicate that the 1x weekly dosing regimen was already administered in a majority of the dialysis patients, when appropriate. The survey was primarily designed to assess current anaemia treatment in Swiss dialysis centres and the relevance of the 1x weekly administration of epoetin beta. Therefore, an open-intervention, practice-based survey design was chosen in order to meet the main objectives. The second objective of this third analysis was to evaluate the efficacy of 1x weekly administration of epoetin beta compared to a more frequent dosing regimen. A randomized clinical study would have been necessary in order to compare the efficacy of two treatment regimens of epoetin beta. Nevertheless, the findings of the survey reveal interesting results about the 1x weekly administration, confirming the efficacy of the 1x weekly administration of previous studies. Such findings have, however, to be interpreted cautiously and are of limited validity.

Haemoglobin levels of the 1x weekly group were comparable to the 2-3x weekly group with no significant difference. A difference of 0.5 g/dl in haemoglobin between the two groups was considered as a normal range of deviation in treatment response to epoetin in dialysis patients and was not considered as a statistical significant difference. This threshold had been previously used in comparable studies [77, 78].

It was expected that a reduction in dosing frequency would lead to a decrease in haemoglobin or that higher epoetin doses were necessary in order to maintain stable haemoglobin levels. In our survey, mean haemoglobin level was equal in both treatment groups. Surprisingly, epoetin beta dose was significantly lower in the 1x weekly group compared to the 2-3x weekly group. Several factors may interfere with the treatment response to epoetin beta and be responsible for higher epoetin dose requirements in the 2-3x weekly group. One responsible factor might be iron deficiency resulting in increased epoetin dose requirements and decreased haemoglobin levels. Iron status was carefully analysed in both groups and was found to be in adherence to the recently published guidelines. The significant difference concerning serum ferritin levels could not explain the increased use of epoetin beta in the 2-3x weekly group, since optimal serum ferritin levels were achieved in both groups. Both groups were well-balanced, since no difference occurred in respect of diagnosis, concomitant diseases, gender and age. One could assume that a higher proportion of epoetin-naïve patients or patients receiving epoetin beta intravenously were included in the 2-3x weekly group which resulted in an increased epoetin dose requirement. The proportion of epoetin-naïve patients was comparable in both groups with no significant difference. Thus, the efficacy of the 1x weekly administration of epoetin beta was analysed in stable dialysis patients (excluding epoetin-naïve patients) and showed a comparable efficacy in both groups with higher epoetin dose requirements in the 2-3x weekly group. The difference in epoetin beta dose between both groups could not be explained by the inclusion of more epoetin-naïve patients. Likewise, the route of administration could not explain the difference in epoetin dose between the two groups. Both groups contained a comparable proportion of patients receiving epoetin beta intravenously and, furthermore, the analyse according to the route of administration showed, that a higher epoetin dose was necessary in the 2-3x weekly than in the 1x weekly group, irrespective of the route of administration.

Other factors may influence epoetin response such as the dialysis quality (Kt/V), the co-medications (ACE inhibitors or AT_1 receptor antagonists), C-reactive protein or iron medications which were not assessed in our survey. It was hypothesized that patients with higher epoetin doses were more likely to receive the weekly epoetin dose divided in 2 or 3 portions, which was confirmed by a univariate analyse. Higher mean weekly epoetin beta dose were more likely to be given as a 2-3x weekly administration and lower epoetin dose were predominately given as a 1x weekly dosing regimen. The 1x weekly administration of epoetin beta was shown to be feasible and efficacious in most dialysis patients, offering beneficial advantages for patients and for medical staff.

The mortality rate of dialysis patients included in "AIMS" was 3.8% after six months and was comparable to the six-month mortality rate of 4.8% found in the "ESAM" survey, conducted in 14 European countries in 1998 and 1999 [119]. One-year survival probability of dialysis patients in the US was 79.2% (one-year survival probability of incident dialysis patients, adjusted, year 2000) [30] and in Europe, 90-day and one-year survival probability of incident dialysis patients (cohort 1993-1997) was 93.6% and 81.4% according to the ERA-EDTA registry report of 2002 [28]. The one-year mortality rate in the Lombardy Dialysis registry (calendar year 1996) was 11.1% and lower than the one reported by the ERA-EDTA registry data base or in the US. One-year mortality rate in "AIMS" is estimated to figure in approximately the similar range as reported by the Lombardy registry. Overall mortality rate was reduced in dialysis patients over time, but the poor long-term survival of ESRD patients is still a matter of concern. Expected life-times for dialysis patients are one third to one sixth of the general population and survival prognoses of patients on dialysis are 2-3x lower than those of transplanted patients [30, 126]. Mortality of patients in "AIMS" was analysed at different thresholds of haemoglobin concentrations, since a more favourable survival probability was expected at higher haemoglobin levels. However, the number of patients and the observation period was not sufficient in order to detect differences in survival at different haemoglobin levels. Morbidities and hospitalization were not assessed in our survey. These parameters would have enabled to investigate the potential association between haemoglobin and morbidity/hospitalization, since large studies have demonstrated an inverse relationship between haemoglobin levels and morbidity/hospitalization rate [96, 97, 146].

In conclusion, the findings show that anaemia of a large proportion of dialyzed patients can be effectively managed with a 1x weekly administration of epoetin beta with a favourable safety profile. The 1x weekly administration results in a decreased number of injections, a higher patient convenience and a reduced workload for nurses and physicians. The easier dosing regimen may also encourage CAPD patients or pre-dialysis patients for self-administration and increase compliance, which may influence the long-term outcome of chronic kidney disease patients.

7. Individualizing anaemia management in dialysis patients in Switzerland – Do co-morbidities and patients' health influence physicians' target haemoglobin?

N. Lötscher[1,2], D. Teta[3], D. Kiss[4], P.-Y. Martin[5], L. Gabutti[6], M. Burnier[3*]

1 Roche (Pharma) Switzerland Ltd, P.O. Box, CH-4153 Reinach, Switzerland
2 Swiss Tropical Institute, Department of Public Health and Epidemiology, P.O. Box, CH-4002 Basel, Switzerland
3 CHUV, Department of Internal Medicine, Nephrology, P.O. Box, CH-1011 Lausanne, Switzerland
4 Kantonsspital Liestal, Department of Nephrology, P.O. Box, CH-4410 Liestal, Switzerland
5 HCUG, Department of Internal Medicine, Nephrology, P.O. Box, CH-1211 Geneva, Switzerland
6 Ospedale regionale La Carità, Department of Nephrology, P.O. Box, CH-6601 Locarno, Switzerland

*Corresponding author:

Tel.: +41 21 314 11 54
E-mail: michel.burnier@hospvd.ch

Working paper to be submitted

7.1 Abstract

Aim: The purpose of the fourth analysis of the "AIMS" survey (*A*naem*I*a *M*anagement in dialysis patients in *S*witzerland) was to assess the prevalence of diagnosis and co-morbidities in dialysis patients in Switzerland compared to US and European databases. The second objective was to assess whether anaemia treatment in dialysis patients was adapted in respect of the co-morbidities of each patient and whether haemoglobin targets were tailored according to the clinical condition of each patient

Method: 368 dialyzed patients of 28 dialysis units in Switzerland were included in this practice-based, open-intervention survey, 340 thereof were eligible. Epidemiological data were collected at baseline and anaemia treatment with epoetin beta was documented over 12 months. The prevalence of diagnosis and co-morbidities of patients included in "AIMS" were evaluated in comparison to the US and ERA-EDTA registry database. Haemoglobin concentration and epoetin beta dose were analyzed according to co-morbidities and diagnosis. Furthermore, a questionnaire was sent to the participating physicians in order to assess target haemoglobin tailored according to the clinical profile of each patient.

Results: The most frequent causes of end-stage renal failure in "AIMS" was glomerulonephritis (23.2%), followed by vascular diseases (21.2%) and diabetes (20.9%). The prevalence of causes of end-stage renal failure corresponded to those of the ERA-EDTA registry database. The most frequent co-morbidities were diabetes (27.4%), coronary artery disease (25.5%) and congestive heart failure (16.5%). Co-morbidities of this survey corresponded as to prevalence to those of the USRDS registry. Mean overall haemoglobin level was 11.8 ±1.0 g/dl and varied between the different co-morbidities. Haemoglobin was highest in COPD (12.2 g/dl) and lowest in heart failure patients (11.4 g/dl). Patients with anaemia of chronic disease (cancer 198 IU/kg/week), heart failure (170 IU/kg/week) and hepatological disorders (191 IU/kg/week) required elevated epoetin dose. Diabetes and heart failure was found to have a significant influence on epoetin dose requirements and haemoglobin and glomerulonephritis on epoetin dose, which was proven by a univariate analysis and a multivariate analysis following thereafter. About 40% of the dialysis centres said to adapt target haemoglobin according to the underlying disease. Two centres individualized target haemoglobin according to the physical conditions of each patient.

Conclusions: Main diagnosis and concomitant diseases of Swiss dialysis patients corresponded in prevalence to the ERA-EDTA and the US registry. A high quality in anaemia management of dialysis patients was achieved in Swiss dialysis. About 40% of all centres adapt target haemoglobin according to the clinical profile of each patient. The EBPG recommend tailoring haemoglobin according to the individual patients, however, well-defined criteria have to be established.

Key words: Anaemia, anaemia management, epoetin, epoetin beta, dosing frequency, end-stage renal disease, European Best Practice Guidelines, EBPG, USRDS, ERA-EDTA, diagnosis, concomitant disease, co-morbidity, comparison

7.2 Introduction

The survey on *A*naem*I*a *M*anagement in dialysis patients in *S*witzerland "AIMS" was designed to assess current anaemia management and co-morbidities in dialysis patients in Switzerland. In a first analysis of the survey, we assessed anaemia management of dialysis patients over a time period of six months in Switzerland, presented in section 4 page 54. In a second analysis, the findings of the first analysis were compared to the current guidelines. The findings showed that anaemia management was well controlled in dialysis patients in Switzerland and approximately 80% of the patients reached target haemoglobin levels of 11 g/dl as recommended by the current guidelines for patients with renal failure. Mean haemoglobin concentration of dialysis patients in Switzerland improved from 11.4 g/dl in 1998 (ESAM trial) [119] to 11.8 g/dl achieved in "AIMS". The ongoing scientific discussion about the optimal haemoglobin level and beneficial outcomes of increasing haemoglobin in dialysis patients might have influenced physicians' target for anaemia treatment towards normalized haemoglobin concentrations in dialysis patients. In this analysis, we assessed the prevalence of causes and concomitant diseases of our population and whether co-morbidities and patients' health influence physicans' target haemoglobin.

Chronic kidney disease is mostly associated with numerous concomitant diseases such as anaemia, diabetes or cardiovascular diseases. Cardiovascular complications are the most frequent cause of death in dialysis patients, accounting for 40% of deaths in these patients [1]. Anaemia itself is an independent risk factor for left ventricular hypertrophy and cardiovascular complications in chronic kidney disease patients, it increases morbidity and mortality [3, 148]. The optimum target haemoglobin concentration for chronic kidney disease patients on erythropoietin treatment is still not fully elucidated, despite the publication of the revised EBPG. Several studies demonstrated that a haemoglobin correction up to a level of 12 g/dl reduced hospitalization rate and mortality and improved quality of life [12, 97, 146, 149]. Patients with congestive heart failure were found to benefit from the anaemia correction (Hb >12g/dl), resulting in improved cardiac function and a lower one-year death rate [120]. In contrast, the study of Besarab et al. was interrupted because total mortality in patients with severe cardiovascular disease was higher in the patient group with normalized haemoglobin levels compared to the patient group with target haemoglobin concentration of 11 g/dl. Based on this controversial evidence, the revised EBPG recommend to keep target haemoglobin between 11 and 12 g/dl for patients with severe cardiovascular disease, unless angina or other symptoms dictate otherwise [82]. For diabetic patients, no controlled data exist to determine the optimal target haemoglobin concentration. As diabetic patients have different blood rheology and mostly suffer from peripheral vascular disease, the EBPG recommend to be cautious and to increase haemoglobin to levels not higher than 12 g/dl. Up to now, only one study has demonstrated beneficial effect of normalized haemoglobin level in diabetes patients [150]. Two large ongoing studies are investigating potential cardiovascular benefits of early normalization of haemoglobin in chronic kidney disease patients (*C*ardiovascular *R*isk Reduction by *E*arly *A*naemia *T*reatment with *E*poetin beta (CREATE) trial) and in diabetes patients with diabetic nephropathy (the *A*naemia *COR*rection in *D*iabetes (Acord) trial). The clinical evidence of the optimal target haemoglobin level in general and in respect of co-morbidities is still unclear, even though some studies indicated beneficial effect in raising haemoglobin level above 12 g/dl. Furthermore, the discussion was held concerning individualizing anaemia treatment in dialysis patients; the target haemoglobin level should be tailored according to the clinical profile of each patient. The revised guidelines recommend target haemoglobin concentrations of ≥11g/dl which should be definded for each individual patient, taking into account gender, age activity and co-morbid conditions. For the first time, guidelines recommend to tailor the target haemoglobin level individually from 11 g/dl to as high as 14 g/dl [82]. To examine this issue further, we analysed achieved mean haemoglobin concentrations in respect of the most common co-morbidities. Each participating dialysis centre was asked whether anaemia treatment in dialysis patients was individualized according to the patients' clinical profile and co-morbidities.

In the present article, as a primary objective we assessed the prevalence of causes and co-morbidities in dialysis patients in Switzerland. As a second objective we investigated whether anaemia treatment in dialysis patients was adapted in respect of the clinical condition of each patient and the implementation of this new treatment strategy postulated by the revised EBPG in dialysis centres in Switzerland, which recommend individualizing anaemia treatment.

7.3 Subjects and methods

Methods

Data used for the fourth analysis derived from the "AIMS" (*A*naem*I*a *M*anagement in dialysis patients in *S*witzerland) survey, a prospective, open-intervention, practice-based survey performed in adult dialysis patients in Switzeralnd. Prevalence of diagnosis and co-morbidities was assessed as well as its influence on aneamia treatment.

Patient recruitment lasted from June 2002 until December 2003 with an observation period of 12 months. The survey did not require any deviation from medical routine as it was practice-based. No approval of the ethical committees is needed for practical-based surveys. 368 dialysis patients of 28 dialysis centres were included, 340 thereof were eligible. Inclusion criteria were dialysis patients (≥ 18 years old) either on haemodialysis or peritoneal dialysis with presence of renal anaemia and being under epoetin therapy or epoetin-naïve. Exclusion criteria were defined according to the contraindication of the product information of epoetin beta and included patients with unstable angina pectoris, untreated hypertension, haemoglobinopathy, haemolysis, epilepsy, pregnancy or lactation. Patients had to be iron-replete (≥ 200 µg/l) and without any deficiency of vitamin B_{12} or folic acid.

At patient registration (baseline), aetiology of chronic renal failure, concomitant diseases, dialysis modality, dry weight and laboratory parameters, such as haemoglobin, serum ferritin, transferrin saturation and serum creatinine were registered. A possible choice of the most common diagnosis (diabetic nephropathy, glomerulonephritis, pyelonephritis/interstitial nephritis) and co-morbidities (coronary artery disease, heart failure, diabetes, hypertension, and blood pressure) was already provided within the report form. Additionally, the physicians had the opportunity to specify the causes and the co-morbidities of the selected patients in a separate row, indicated as others. Laboratory parameters were documented if performed in the course of the clinical routine. Epoetin beta treatment (weekly dose, frequency and route of administration) and haemoglobin concentration were monthly assessed. The received filled-in data report forms were examined on completeness of mandatory data and validated prior to data entry. Data were defined as mandatory for dry weight, haemoglobin, dosage and frequency of epoetin beta treatment. Patients were included if they fulfilled the inclusion criteria.

In this article, the prevalence of diagnosis and co-morbidities of dialysis patients were analysed as a primary goal. Epidemiological data of Swiss dialysis patients, based on the "AIMS" survey, were compared to international registry data of dialysis patients from the US and Europe. For this purpose, reported diagnoses were clustered into diagnosis groups according to the US diagnosis categories. The second objective was to assess whether co-morbidities and patients' physical condition influence haemoglobin concentration. Haemoglobin concentrations were analysed per co-morbidity and their influence on aneamia treatment was assessed in a univariate and multivariate analysis. Furthermore, it was assessed whether physicians tailor target haemoglobin according to co-morbid and physical condition of each patient. This information was gathered on a separate questionnaire assessing physicians' target haemoglobin levels in respect of the patients' co-morbid condition. All participating dialysis centres were asked to fill in this questionnaire. For the questionnaire see Appendix II.

Statistical analysis

All statistical tests were performed using SAS, version 8.1 (SAS Institute, Cary, NC, USA), Excel 2002 or Epi-Info®, version 3.2. Last observation carried forward method (LOCF) was used for value replacement. Standard descriptive statistics were calculated for the patients' age, gender, co-morbidities, and diagnosis and baseline laboratory parameters. Diagnosis and co-morbidities data of the dialysis patients included in "AIMS" were characterized and compared to the US and European regristry using descriptive statistics. Point prevalence were calculated for diagnosis and co-morbidities of ESRD at patient registration (=baseline). All prevalence data are unadjusted data for age and gender. Descriptive statistics were used to analyse anaemia treatment in Swiss dialysis centres including 95% confidence interval, mean, median and standard deviation for the primary variables (haemoglobin and epoetin beta dose). Categorical variables were compared using the χ^2-test and continuous variables using Students' t-test, Wilcoxon two-sample and Kruskal-Wallis test, where appropriate. Univariate analyse was performed for haemoglobin and epoetin beta dose regarding concomitant disease, diagnosis, age and gender. A multivariate analyse was performed which included only the covariates with p <0.05 in the univeriate analyse. All statistical tests were two-sided and the significance was tested on a 0.05 p value.

7.4 Results

7.4.1 Patient characteristics

Six months data are presented in this article. The analysis was performed on 340 eligible dialysis patients, 95% thereof were on haemodialysis and 5% on peritoneal dialysis. 18 of 340 patients were epoetin-naïve patients. A detailed overview of the treatment population is given in section 3.8.1 page 46.

58.2% of the patients were male and 41.8% female. Demographic characteristics of the studied population demonstrate that most patients (male and female) on dialysis are at middle or at advanced age. Mean age was 63.5 ± 14.7 years, ranging from 18 to 91. More than 70% of the patients were older than 60 years. Mean age for males and females were 63.8 ± 14.3 years and 63.1 ± 27.7 years (p=0.62, Students' t-test). Baseline haemoglobin concentration was 11.8 ± 1.4 g/dl, ranging from 6.8-15.5 (95% CI 11.6-11.9). Demographics and diagnosis of ESRD are described in section 3.8.2, page 47. In brief, glomerulonephritis (23.2%) was the most common cause of ESRD, followed by diabetic nephropathy (20.9%), hypertension and vascular disease (21.2%). Polycystic kidney disease (7.9%) and tumours (2.6%) were less frequent causes of ESRD.

7.4.2 Prevalence of causes and co-morbidities in dialysis patients in Switzerland

Diagnosis

The causes of dialysis patients in "AIMS" were comparable to the US [1] and European registry data [126] with some differences, as illustrated in Table 7-1. Glomerulonephritis, hypertension and vascular causes were the most frequent diagnosis in Swiss dialysis patients reported in "AIMS", followed by diabetic nephropathy with 21%. The prevalence of diabetic nephropathy was 1.7 fold higher in the US (36%, USRDS) than reported in "AIMS" (21%) and occurred less frequently in Europe (13%, ERA-EDTA). Diabetes was the main cause for ESRD in elderly patients according to the USRDS registry [1].

These findings were confirmed in "AIMS". The relative risk of diabetes was 2.9 fold higher in patients older than 50 years compared to younger patients (CI 1.2-6.9) (p=0.007; χ^2-test). The prevalence of glomerulonephritis was comparable between "AIMS" and the ERA-EDTA registry and was observed more often in younger patients. Glomerulonephritis was less frequently reported (14.5%) in incident patients in the US than in Europe (data not shown) [30].

Diagnosis	USRDS 2004 annual report (prevalence data, December 2002)[1]		ERA-EDTA registry (prevalence data, December 2002)[2]		CH ("AIMS" survey)	
	n	%	n	%	n*	%
Diabetic nephropathy	154,197	35.8	11,566	13.3	71	20.9
Glomerulonephritis	67,207	15.6	20,190	23.2	79	23.2
Pyelonephritis / interstitial nephritis	n.n.[3]	n.n.[3]	10,196	11.7	58	17.1
Hypertension / renal vascular disease	102,385	23.7	9,469	10.9	72	21.2
Polycystic kidney disease (PKD)	18,560	4.3	7,778	8.9	27	7.9
Unclear	15,875	3.7	14,378	16.5	13	3.8
Miscellaneous causes	52,551	12.2	13,405	15.4	19	5.6
Missing diseases	6,212	1.4	--	--	9	2.8

[1] Prevalent counts of reported ESRD patients, patients alive on 31 December 2002, by primary diagnosis [30]
[2] Prevalence per million population and percentage, unadjusted. Prevalent patients on December 31 (2002), by cause of renal failure [28]
[3] Incidence of reported ESRD, 1998-2002 combined, according to USRDS: Interstitial nephritis/pyelonephritis: 17,579 patients (3.8%), as of December 2002
*Naming of one or more diagnosis per patient was possible; therefore the figures are not cumulative. n.n = not named

Table 7-1: Diagnoses of ESRD in the US, in Europe and in "AIMS"

Table 7-2 provides an overview of registered diagnoses of end-stage renal diseases per country as reported to the ERA-EDTA registry.

Prevalence data of diagnoses of ESRD as of 31 December, 2002 are presented in % of all countries reporting to the ERA-EDTA registry. A high variability of primary causes of ESRD occurred between the ERA-EDTA reporting countries for diabetic nephropathy, hypertension and renal vascular disease (RVD). The prevalence of pyelonephritis was comparable in all ERA-EDTA reporting countries. Diabetic nephropathy occurred more frequently in Austria, Sweden and Finland than in Spain and the Netherlands. The prevalence of glomerulonephritis was higher in northern European countries (Norway and Sweden) than in southern European countries. Hypertension and renal vascular disease were the most frequent cause of ESRD, highest in Iceland followed by Switzerland (patients of "AIMS"). In other ERA-EDTA reporting countries hypertension and renal vascular disease were less frequently reported causes of ESRD.

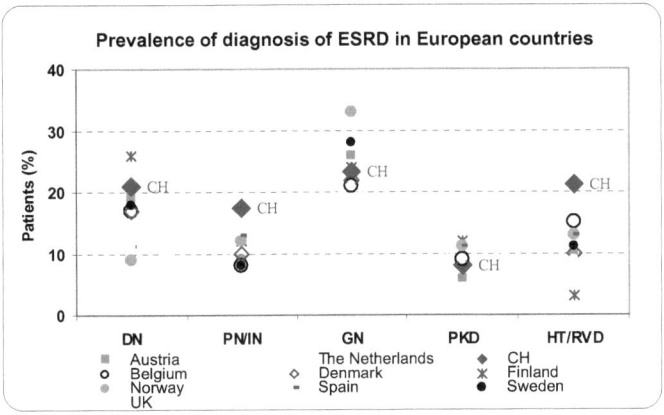

Diagnosis of ESRD of ERA-EDTA country (in %)	DN	PN	GN	PKD	HT / RVD	Misc	Unknown
Austria	19	9	26	6	10	18	11
Belgium, Dutch-speaking	17	8	21	9	15	21	10
Denmark	17	10	22	8	10	16	17
Finland	26	12	24	12	3	18	6
Greece	15	8	23	8	10	8	27
Iceland	7	13	21	6	24	25	5
Norway	9	12	33	11	13	19	3
Spain, Catalonia	11	13	23	11	13	10	19
Spain, Valencia	9	14	20	9	16	11	22
Sweden	18	8	28	9	11	20	6
The Netherlands	9	12	21	8	13	18	18
UK	11	14	21	9	9	15	19
Diagnosis of ESRD of non-ERA-EDTA country							
CH (findings of "AIMS")	21	17	23	8	21	4	3

DN=diabetic nephropathy, PN= pyelonephritis, GN=glomerulonephritis, PKD=polycystic kidney disease, HT=hypertension, RVD= renal vascular disease, Misc=miscellaneous

Table 7-2: Prevalence of causes by country

Co-morbidities

Dialysis patients are co-morbid patients. Co-morbidities were reported in 87% of all patients included in "AIMS" and in more than 40% two or more concomitant diseases (cardiovascular diseases or diabetes) were reported. Most frequent co-morbidities of the "AIMS" patients were cardiovascular diseases (47.3%), hypertension (60.6%) and diabetes (27%). The prevalence of coronary artery disease, heart failure and diabetes increased with age and a positive linear relationship was observed between coronary artery disease (r^2=0.889) and age and between heart failure and age (r^2=0.873). The relative risk of coronary artery disease was four times higher in elderly patients than in the younger patient group ($\leq$ 50 years) (p=0.0036, χ^2-test). Coronary artery disease in "AIMS" occurred as frequently as in US end-stage renal disease patients included in the USRDS registry. The prevalence of coronary disease increased proportionally with age and was comparable between patients included in "AIMS" and the US registry database, as illustrated in Figure 7-1.

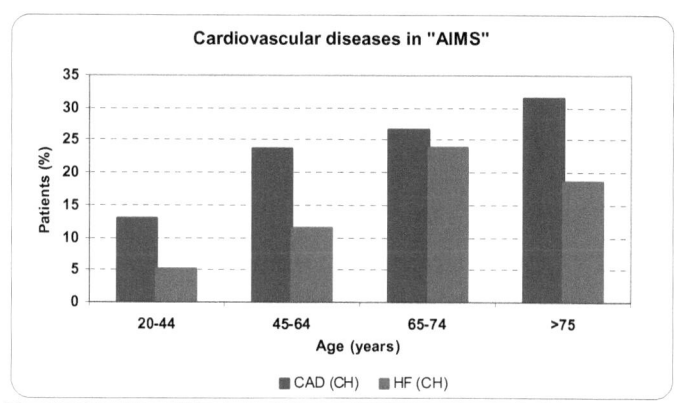

Age (years)	Coronary artery disease, in %	
	"AIMS"	USRDS 2004[1]
20-44	12.8	4.6
45-64	23.6	20.6
65-74	26.6	32.8
>75	31.4	35.6

[1] USRDS 2004 annual report (Diseases of incident ESRD patients, 2002) [30]

Figure 7-1: Cardiovascular diseases of ESRD patients reported in "AIMS" and in USRDS

Congestive heart failure was reported in twice as many patients in the US as in patients included in our survey (31.7 % versus 16.5%). Table 7-3 shows a comparison of diagnoses between "AIMS" data and the USRDS report.

Overview of most frequently reported cardiovascular diseases (in %)	"AIMS"	USRDS[1]
Coronary artery disease	25.5	24.9
Congestive heart failure	16.5	31.1
Hypertension	60.6	79.3
Vascular diseases	5.0	13.9
COPD	1.8	7.6
Cancer	2.0	6.2

[1] USRDS 2004 annual report (Diseases of incident ESRD patients, 2002) [30]

Table 7-3: Overview of concomitant diseases in the US and in "AIMS"

7.4.3 Influence of co-morbidities on haemoglobin and physicians' target haemoglobin

Influence of co-morbid conditions on haemoglobin concentration

Mean haemoglobin levels were comparable for all concomitant pathologies and were on average above the EBPG recommendations. Some variation had been observed considering minimum and maximum levels. Mean haemoglobin was highest in patients with COPD (Hb=12.2 ± 1.0 g/dl) and lowest in patients with hyperparathyroidism (Hb=11.4 ± 0.6 g/dl). Mean haemoglobin concentration in patients with diabetes was 12.0 ± 1.0 g/dl and in patients with cardiovascular diseases, it ranged between 11.5 and 11.8 g/dl. Mean haemoglobin level was below average (overall mean Hb: 11.8 ± 1.0 g/dl) in patients with heart failure (11.5 ± 1.0 g/dl), with cancer (11.5 ± 0.9 g/dl), with hyperparathyroidism (11.4 ±0.6 g/dl) and with hepatological disorders (11.6 ±1.3 g/dl). Mean haemoglobin level of patients with diabetes and coronary artery disease was comparable to the overall average haemoglobin, as illustrated in Figure 7-2. The influence of the underlying concomitant disease on the haemoglobin concentration was investigated in a univariate analysis. Significant higher haemoglobin concentrations were achieved in patients with diabetes (p=0.02) and significantly lower haemoglobin concentrations in patients with heart failure (p=0.04), which was prooven in a second, multivariate analysis. Diabetes was found to influence haemoglobin level significantly towards higher concentration and heart failure towards lower haemoglobin level in dialysis patients. Age, gender and menstruation (females <50 years) were not found to influence haemoglobin level in the univariate analyse.

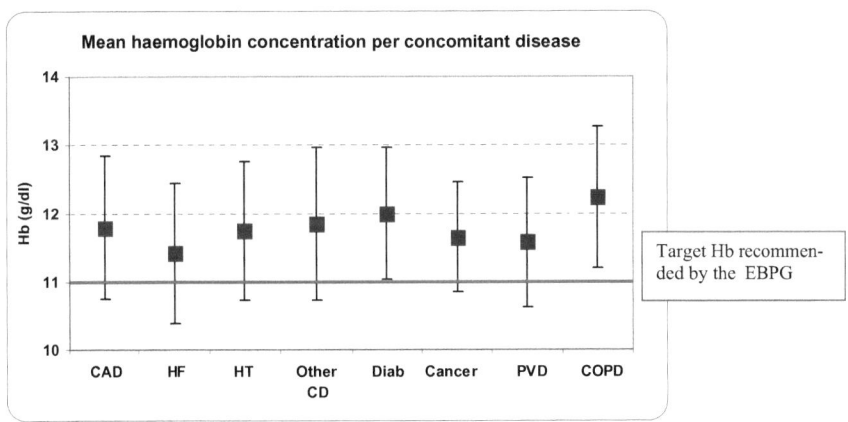

	Total	CAD	HF	HT	Other CD	Diabetes[1]	Cancer[1]	PVD	COPD
Patients	340	87	56	206	18	93	15	72	6
Mean Hb (g/dl)	11.8	11.7	11.5	11.7	11.8	12.0	11.5	11.8	12.2
SD	1.0	1.0	1.0	1.0	1.1	1.0	0.9	1.0	1.0
p value		0.15	0.04	0.4	0.8	0.02	0.2	0.9	0.27

CAD=coronary artery disease; HF=heart failure; HT= hypertension; Other CD=other cardiac diseases; Diab=diabetes; PVD= polyvascular disease; COPD = chronic obstructive pulmonary disease
[1] overall (reported as diagnosis and concomitant disease)

Figure 7-2: Mean haemoglobin by concomitant disease

Figure 7-3 demonstrates the proportion of patients included in "AIMS" with achieved mean haemoglobin levels at thresholds of 11 g/dl and 12 g/dl, respectively, stratified according to concomitant diseases. Mean haemoglobin level was in 87% of all diabetes patients above 11g/dl and no difference was observed between diabetes and non-diabetes patients in respect of the achieved haemoglobin concentration (p=0.1979; χ^2-test). 37.5% of all diabetes patients had a haemoglobin concentration between 11 and 12 g/dl and 46.3% above 12 g/dl. 78% and 35% of the patients with coronary artery disease achieved haemoglobin levels of $\geq$11 g/dl and of $\geq$12 g/dl, respectively. Similarly, in patients with heart failure, 75% and 30% achieved haemoglobin levels of $\geq$11 g/dl and $\geq$12 g/dl, respectively. Fewer patients with cancer and heart failure reached haemoglobin concentrations of 11 g/dl. This was confirmed in a univariate analysis for heart failure solely. Heart failure showed to have a significant influence on haemoglobin concentrations towards lower levels in these patients.

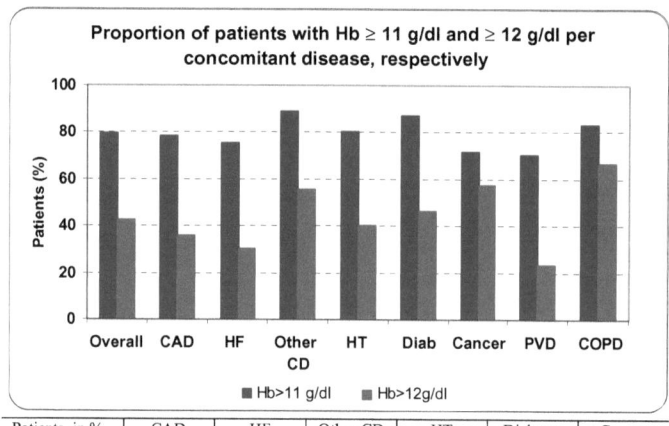

Patients, in %	CAD (n=87)	HF (n=56)	Other CD (n=18)	HT (n=206)	Diabetes (n=93)	Cancer (n=15)
Hb $\geq$ 11 g/dl	78.2	75.0	88.9	80.1	87.1	71.4
Hb $\geq$ 12 g/dl	35.6	30.4	55.6	40.3	46.2	57.1

CAD= coronary artery disease; HF= heart failure; Other CD=other cardiac diseases; HT= hypertension

Figure 7-3: Percentage of patients with Hb>11 g/dl and >12 g/dl, respectively, per concomitant disease

Influence of co-morbid conditions on treatment response to epoetin

Table 7-4 provides a summary of haemoglobin concentrations and administered epoetin beta doses per co-morbidity or cause of CKD. In comparison to the overall mean epoetin beta dose (149 ± 104 IU/kg/week), elevated epoetin beta doses were necessary in tumour patients, in patients with hepatological disorders, heart failure and hyperparathyroidism. Mean weekly epoetin beta dose was 198 ± 138 IU/kg/week in tumour patients with a trend towards higher epoetin dose requirements (p=0.06). Patients with hepatological disorders required elevated but not significantly higher epoetin doses (191 ± 121 IU/kg/week; p=0.2). Mean weekly epoetin dose was elevated in patients with hyperparathyroidism (170 ± 179 IU/kg/week) with a high variation from 30-500 IU/kg/week. A reduced need of epoetin dose was expected in polycystic kidney disease patients, which, though, was not confirmed within this survey. Mean weekly epoetin dose for patients with PKD was 154 ± 124 IU/kg/week. The influence of the underlying disease on haemoglobin level and required epoetin dose was investigated in a univariate and, thereafter, in a multivariate analysis. Diabetes showed to have a significant influence on haemoglobin and epoetin dose requirements, as depicted in Table 7-4.

Significant higher haemoglobin levels were achieved in diabetes patients (p=0.02) with significant lower administered epoetin dosages (p=0.0004). In contrast, significantly lower haemoglobin levels were achieved in patients with heart failure (p=0.04), with a trend towards higher epoetin dose requirements (p=0.098). Glomerulonephritis was found to have a significant influence on the epoetin dose (p=0.048). Tumour patients required elevated epoetin dosages compared to the average, though with no significant difference (p=0.06).

Primary and concomitant diseases		Mean haemoglobin level (g/dl)			Mean weekly epoetin beta dosage (IU/kg/week)		
	Patients (n)	Mean ± SD	Confidence interval	p value	Mean ± SD	Confidence interval	p value
Diabetes[1]	93	12.0 ± 1.0	11.8 – 12.2	0.02	117 ± 68	103 – 131	0.0004
Pyelonephritis / Int. nephritis	58	11.9 ± 1.0	11.6 – 12.1	0.43	137 ± 81	116 – 159	0.34
Glomerulo-nephritis	79	11.7 ± 1.0	11.5 – 12.0	0.67	170 ± 123	142 – 197	0.048
Polyvascular disease	72	11.8 ± 1.0	11.6 – 12.0	0.98	132 ± 82	113 – 152	0.12
Polycystic kidney disease	27	11.9 ± 0.9	11.6 – 12.3	0.43	154 ± 124	105 – 203	0.82
Cancer[2]	15	11.5 ± 0.9	11.0 – 12.0	0.23	198 ± 138	122 – 275	0.06
Coronary artery disease	87	11.7 ± 1.0	11.4 – 11.9	0.15	159 ± 110	136 – 183	0.30
Heart failure	56	11.5 ± 1.0	11.3 – 11.8	0.04	170 ± 130	136 – 205	0.098
Hypertension	206	11.7 ± 1.0	11.6 – 11.9	0.37	143 ± 87	131 – 155	0.15
Other cardiac diseases	18	11.8 ± 1.1	11.3 – 12.4	0.79	158 ± 84	116 – 200	0.72
COPD	6	12.2 ± 1.0	11.2 – 13.2	0.27	155 ± 108	41 – 268	0.89
Hyperpara-thyroidism	6	11.4 ± 0.6	10.7 – 12.0	0.31	170± 179	-18 – 358	0.63
Hepatological disorders	7	11.6 ± 1.3	10.4 – 12.8	0.62	191 ± 121	79 – 303	0.28
Overall	340	11.8 ± 1.0	11.7 – 11.9	-	149 ± 104	138 – 160	-

Multiple entries possible, therefore not cumulative
[1] Diabetes: diabetes reported as concomitant disease (n=79) and/or diagnosis of ESRD (n=75). In 31 patients diabetes was reported as primary cause and concomitant disease; [2] Cancer: co-morbidity (n=7) and diagnosis (n=9)

Table 7-4: Haemoglobin level and mean weekly epoetin beta dose per disease

Do dialysis centres individualize anaemia treatment in respect of the patients' co-morbid condition and health stage?

38.5% (10 of 26 centres) of the centres reported to adapt target haemoglobin levels according to the underlying disease of dialysis patients. The majority of the centres aimed at equal target haemoglobin concentrations for all dialysis patients irrespective of the co-morbidity. Table 7-5 provides an overview of dialysis centres differentiating haemoglobin targets according to the respective co-morbidity. In dialysis centres with individualized anaemia treatment, higher target haemoglobin concentrations were generally aimed at in patients with cardiac diseases, ranging from 11 g/dl to 14 g/dl. Target haemoglobin levels for dialysis patients with coronary artery disease or with heart failure were in 90% of these centres (with indiviual anaemia treatment) above 12 g/dl. Two centres aimed at individual haemoglobin targets for dialysis patients in respect of age, co-morbidities and physical condition. Target haemoglobin concentrations were in all dialysis centres above 11 g/dl and in 58% of the centres above 12 g/dl.

Dialysis centre	Patients	Physicians' target Hb	Tailoring Hb target according to the patients' health and co-morbid condition?	
	n	Target Hb (g/dl)	Co-morbidity	Target Hb (g/dl)
1	3	12	Individual targets (co-morbidity, physical condition, age)	11-13.5
2	5	11.5-12.5	CAD (symptomatic)	12-13
3	23	11-12	CAD, heart failure	12.5-13.5
4	26	11-12	Heart failure, young and sportive, individual targets	> 12
5	13	>11	-	-
6	6	12	CAD (symptomatic)	12-13
7	34	12	Ischaemic cardiomyopathy	≥13
8	16	11-12	-	-
9	19	12	-	-
11	14	12.5	-	-
12	16	12	-	-
13	16	12	CAD (symptomatic)	13
14	20	13 (40%)	-	-
15	2	12	-	-
16	10	11-12	-	-
17	5	11-13	-	-
18	25	13	Coronaropathy, respiratory insufficiency	14
19	8	12-13	CAD (symptomatic)	>12.5
20	10	>11.5	-	-
21	4	12	-	-
22	14	12-13	-	-
23	10	11-12	-	-
24	12	12.5-13.5	-	-
26	10	11.5	-	-
27	9	12	Heart failure (severe)	13
28	10	11-12	-	-

No values for centre 10 and 25 due to study exclusion (missing reports).
-: No individual haemoglobin target

Table 7-5: Overview of achieved mean haemoglobin and centre-specific target haemoglobin levels

7.5 Discussion

The analysis showed that the frequency of diagnosis and co-morbidities in dialysis patients in "AIMS" were comparable to those of the USRDS and the European registry database with some deviations. The prevalence of diabetic nephropathy and congestive heart failure was higher in the US than in patients of the "AIMS" survey. The majority of the dialysis patients suffered from at least one or more co-morbidities with highest prevalence for diabetes and cardiac diseases. Mean haemoglobin concentrations varied between the different co-morbidities and were highest in patients with COPD and lowest in cancer patients. Administered epoetin dose was highest in cancer patients. Diabetes and heart failure showed to have a significant influence on haemoglobin and epoetin dose. Glomerulonephritis was found to have a significant influence on the epoetin dose requirements. About 40% of all dialysis centres adapted haemoglobin according to the underlying co-morbidity. The majority of the dialysis centres aimed at identical haemoglobin targets for all dialysis patients and did not tailor anaemia treatment in respect of the patients' co-morbidity and physical health.

The comparison of the findings in "AIMS" with international registries in terms of diagnosis and co-morbidities may further support the validity of our survey. The ERA-EDTA registry is the European renal registry database, with 15 national and regional European registries providing annually individual patient data. The USRDS database contains all Medicare payment data and, consequently, data of almost all end-stage renal disease patients in the US are available. Both registries contain combined aetiology data of all end-stage renal disease patients (dialysis and transplanted patients), "AIMS", however, included solely dialysis patients. Therefore the question could be raised to know whether the prevalence data of "AIMS" was comparable to those registries. Since the proportion of transplanted patients in respect of the total end-stage renal population was small, aetiologies and co-morbidities of ESRD were not expected to change considerably for dialysis patients. A descriptive comparison of registries might provide interesting epidemiological information, however the findings have to be interpreted cautiously, since the classifications of certain criteria (disease categories, data analysis and presentation) may vary between the different sources.

Main diagnoses of Swiss dialysis patients corresponded to those of the ERA-EDTA reporting countries. Differencies occurred in the frequency of certain aetiologies between "AIMS" and the USRDS registry database [126]. Glomerulonephritis was the most frequent cause of ESRD in "AIMS", followed by hypertension and diabetic nephropathy. In contrast, diabetes was the most common cause attributed to ESRD in the US, followed by hypertension and glomerulonephritis [1, 2, 126]. Diabetes was one of the most increasing causes of ESRD, representing 45% and 24% of all incident patients in the US and in Europe, respectively. It will still raise in future, due to the sharp increase in prevalence of type 2 diabetes in industrialized countries which is a consequence of the overnutrition and the increasing prevalence of adipositas [151, 152]. A higher variation in prevalence was observed for renal vascular disease between the different European countries (4% in Finland and 36% in Iceland) and US (24%). This can be explained by the fact that the causality between hypertension and primary cause for ESRD is very difficult to be prooven. While the attribution of ESRD to diseases such as diabetes and polycystic kidney disease is quite certain, other causes of ESRD such as hypertension might be more difficult to ascribe and may explain certain discrepancies. The greatest differences between the registries occurred in the prevalence of diabetes and renal vascular disease, which are the leading and still increasing causes of end-stage renal disease.

Dialysis patients are multi-morbid patients. Most common co-morbidities were hypertension and cardiac-related diseases. Coronary artery disease is very common in dialysis patients and its presence is a predictor for a shortened life span. Coronary artery disease occurred in one fourth of all patients included in "AIMS" and its prevalence was comparable to those of the US registry [1], the ESAM survey [119] and the European-DOPPS study [146]. The Dialysis Morbidity and Mortality study Wave 2 (DMMS Wave 2), however, reported a higher frequency of coronary artery disease in dialysis patients (40%) [130]. The reasons for the differences between the DMMS study and the USRDS registry could not be explained by the authors of the DMMS study. Congestive heart failure occurred in the US in twice as many patients as in "AIMS". This difference might be explainable by the selected survey method (practice-based, open-intervention) and it could be hypothesized that co-morbidities were not reported for all patients in "AIMS".

In the recently publisd European-DOPPS study [146] and the ESAM survey [119] congestive heart failure occurred in 25% (range: 12% in Italy; 33% in UK) and 15% of the included patients, respectively, thus confirming the findings of "AIMS". These data are more likely to suggest that differences exist in the occurrence of congestive heart failure between US and European end-stage renal failure patients. The prevalence of congestive heart failure in "AIMS" corresponded to the European-DOPPS study and the ESAM survey, which counterbalanced the risk of underreporting in "AIMS". The data reflect a high prevalence of cardiovascular co-morbidities in dialysis patients which increased by age and thus influenced survival importantly.

Anaemia treatment was analysed in respect of the co-morbidities. The findings suggest that haemoglobin was well controlled in patients with co-morbidities and was above the recommendations of the EBPG postulating target haemoglobin levels of ≥ 11 g/dl for dialysis patients. Mean haemoglobin concentration was highest in patients with chronic obstructive pulmonary disease and lowest in heart failure and cancer patients. Elevated epoetin beta doses were needed in patients with cancer, hepatological disorders, heart failure and hyperparathyroidism. Diabetes patients achieved significantly higher haemoglobin levels (12 g/dl), which figured in the upper range of the EBPG guidelines. Approximately half of all diabetes patients achieved haemoglobin of >12 g/dl, indicating a gap between the EBPG recommendations and clinical practice in Switzerland. Heart failure patients however required considerably higher epoetin doses with significantly lower achieved haemoglobin levels.

Mean haemoglobin level of heart failure patients was in adherence to the EBPG guidelines, which recommend to keep patients with severe cardiovascular diseases at a haemoglobin level of 11-12 g/dl [82]. The basis of this recommendation was set by the United States Normal Hematocrit Trial where a significant higher death rate and occurrence of myocard infarctions was observed in the normalized haematocrit group [115].

While haemoglobin concentration corresponded to the recommendation, a higher epoetin dose was necessary in CHF patients compared to average. Severe congestive heart failure can further exacerbate anaemia as cytokines are released by the damaged myocard, which can further damage heart and kidney and therefore worsen anaemia [153]. This might explain the increased epoetin requirements of patients with heart failure and the considerably lower response to anaemia treatment. This vicious circle is called the cardio-renal syndrome [121, 154]. Silverberg et al. showed in a study with congestive heart failure patients that the prevalence of anaemia increased with the severity of cardiac failure, and treatment with epoetin improved cardiac and renal function in these patients

[120]. Chronic kidney disease patients with severe congestive heart failure were shown to benefit from target haemoglobin levels of 12 or 12.5 g/dl compared to the lower haemoglobin levels (Hb: 10.3 g/dl), which resulted in an improved LVEF, NYHA class and a reduced number of hospitalization days [120]. Overall, these findings suggest that anaemia correction is beneficial to those patients, particularly in respect of cardiomyopathy. However, further trials are necessary in order to confirm whether a physiologically targeted approach can improve clinical coutcome.

Patients with solid tumour and multiple myeloma require generally higher epoetin doses in order to response to anaemia treatment [155-157]. There was a trend towards higher epoetin dose in tumour patients compared to the overall population in "AIMS". Responsible factors for poorer epoetin response in those patients might be bone marrow infiltration by tumour cells and chemotherapy, beside inflammatory processes and cytokines, which inhibit erythropoietin production and iron utilization [158, 159]. There appear similarities in anaemia between cancer patients and chronic kidney disease patients, where inflammatory factors (cytokines, tumour necrosis factors) have a negative impact on the differentiation of erythroid precursors and on the response to erythropoietin [160].

Responsible factors for elevated epoetin dose requirements in hepatological disorders might be the presence of pro-inflammatory cytokines due to inflammation processes which can negatively influence the maturation of red cell precursors, leading thus to anaemia and hyporesponsiveness to epoetin treatment [56, 161]. Hyperparathyroidism and histological osteitis fibrosis are often associated with resistance to the action of epoetin. The excessive secretion of parathyroid hormone leads to bone marrow fibrosis and, consequently, to interference with erythropoiesis. In our survey, elevated mean weekly epoetin doses were required in patients with hyperparathyroidism with a high interpatient-variation. The stage of bone marrow fibrosis or osteitis differs in those patients in respect of the degree of osseous effects of the parathyroid hormone, which might explain the high variation of epoetin administration in hyperparathyroid patients [54, 55, 162, 163]. Polycystic kidney disease patients require generally smaller epoetin doses due to their residual endogenous erythropoietin production. This was not be confirmed by the results of "AIMS", where mean epoetin dose and haemoglobin of polycystic kidney disease patients corresponded to the average values of the total survey population.

The available guidelines for anaemia management are evidence-based and provide guidance in the treatment of anaemia in chronic kidney disease patients, but the question about the optimal target haemoglobin concentration still remains unanswered. The recommended target haemoglobin concentrations may not be appropriate for all patients and may need to be adapted individually. 40% of the participating centres said to tailor haemoglobin concentration according to the underlying co-morbidity, particularly in the case of heart failure or symptomatic coronary artery disease. Few centres took into account other factors such as gender, age and physical condition when deciding on the target haemoglobin. The recently issued revised EBPG recommend to individualize and to tailor anaemia treatment according to the clinical profile of each patient, yet they do not explain how nor do they provide specific criterias.

Anaemia management in patients included in the "AIMS" survey was well controlled and above the recommendations of the guidelines. Despite this fact, less than half of the centres tailored anaemia treatment in dialysis patients in respect of the co-morbidity and the patients' clinical profile. The implementation of these new treatment strategies will require more time. However, it is more important that the EBPG define target haemoglobin levels for individual patient groups. Therefore, more appropriate evidence-based guidelines and well-defined criteria have to be established in further trials in order to individualize renal anaemia management.

8. Conclusions and recommendations

8.1 Background and objectives

*A*naem*I*a *M*anagement of dialysis patients in *S*witzerland "AIMS" was the first survey performed in Switzerland assessing the clinical practice of anaemia treatment in Swiss dialysis patients after the edition of the European Best Practice Guidelines (EBPG) in 1998. The guidelines were issued with the objective to provide European nephrologists evidence-based recommendations for the anaemia treatment in chronic kidney disease patients in order to improve and optimize patient care. Current practice of anaemia correction aims at partial normalization and the guidelines recommend target haemoglobin levels higher than 11 g/dl. The European Survey in Anaemia Management (ESAM), however, gave evidence that the modest targets recommended by the guidelines were not achieved in a great majority of dialysis patients.

Over the last decade, new findings have successively influenced anaemia treatment of chronic kidney disease patients. Epoetin was first administered 3-7 times a week intravenously and then predominately used for subcutaneous administration, since several studies demonstrated a greater efficacy of the subcutaneous administration, thus allowing to further increase the dosing interval. Despite the long experience in the field of anaemia management the optimum target haemoglobin level with the most beneficial outcome for patients with chronic kidney disease has not yet been defined. Revised guidelines even recommend to tailor target haemoglobin levels according to the clinical profile of each patient; still, they do not specify targets for individual patient groups. Out of this unclear situation regarding the optimum target haemoglobin concentration, the following question arised: What is the clinical practice of anaemia management in Swiss dialysis centres today and does anaemia treatment adhere to the current guidelines? In order to answer specifically to these questions, the survey was designed to assess the following objectives:

The first objective consisted in investigating the current clinical practice of anaemia treatment in dialysis patients cared in Swiss dialysis centres. The second objective was to compare the achieved findings to the current guidelines in order to assess the adherence of anaemia treatment in Switzerland to the EBPG. In a third analysis, we evaluated the relevance of the 1x weekly administration of epoetin beta in dialysis patients, given the fact that there was still limited experience since the European approval in 2001. The fourth objective should assess whether nephrologists tailored anaemia treatment according to the clinical condition of each patient. Furthermore, we evaluated the influence of co-morbidities on haemoglobin and epoetin dose.

8.2 Methodology

The "AIMS" survey was a prospective, practice-based, open-intervention survey (clinical reports, Praxiserfahrungsbericht) designed to assess current anaemia management in dialysis centres in Switzerland.

As patients are not directly accessible, dialysis centres were contacted in order to include the respective target population. A higher participation rate as well as a better representativity were expected by contacting all dialysis centres instead of selecting dialysis centres randomly. Therefore, all dialysis centres in Switzerland were contacted in June 2002 and asked for their participation in the survey. After positive consent of the dialysis centre, dialysis patients were consecutively recruited by the responsible medical person. Concerning the dialysis patients, fulfilling of the inclusion and exclusion criteria and the baseline parameters were documented in the pre-printed clinical report forms. Anaemia treatment was monthly documented during an observation period of 12 months. At survey interruption, the final report form was asked to be completed by stating the reasons for discontinuation. Serious adverse events occuring in relation with epoetin beta were requested to be documented in a separate spontaneous adverse event form. A separate questionnaire was sent to all participating dialysis centres in order to assess whether target haemoglobin was tailored according to the patients' health and co-morbid stage.

368 dialysis patients were included in the survey deriving from 28 Swiss dialysis centres, corresponding to 40% of the total number of dialysis centres. The high proportion of included patients (10% of the total Swiss dialysis population) and the good coverage allowed to draw reasonable conclusions about the current anaemia management in dialysis patients in Switzerland. Thus, the included dialysis patients in "AIMS" were representative for the total dialysis population in Switzerland, as discussed in section 3.7, page 43. Further evidence was given by the fact that the prevalence of co-morbidities and diagnosis in our survey corresponded to the prevalence in European countries reporting to the ERA-EDTA registry.

8.3 Key results and lessons learnt

The findings of the first six months were presented in this thesis revealing new insights into renal anaemia management in Switzerland. The findings of "AIMS" suggest that a high quality of anaemia management was achieved in a great majority of dialysis patients cared in Swiss dialysis centres. Mean haemoglobin concentration was 11.8 g/dl at month 6 with 80% of the included patients achieving the target haemoglobin level of ≥ 11 g/dl recommended by the EBPG. Haemoglobin concentrations improved over the last five years in Switzerland and were higher than in most other European countries [28, 119]. Mean epoetin beta dose was 149 IU/kg/week and figured in the upper range of the target of 50-150 IU/kg/week recommended by the EBPG, which is explainable by the fact that higher haemoglobin levels are generally associated with increased epoetin dose.

Anaemia management in Swiss dialysis centres was mostly in adherence to the EBPG. Target haemoglobin levels of most dialysis centres were even higher than recommended by the guidelines. More than 80% of the participating physicians aimed at haemoglobin levels of 12 g/dl or higher, whereof nearly one fourth of them even aimed at full normalization (≥ 13 g/dl) in dialysis patients. Physicians' target haemoglobin was achieved in only 48% of the patients compared to 80% achieving 11 g/dl, since physicians' goals were more ambitious with a tendency to normalized haemoglobin concentrations. 40% of all dialysis centres said to adapt target haemoglobin concentrations according to co-morbidities and the physical condition of each patient. The majority of the dialysis centres, however, aimed at identical target haemoglobin concentrations for all dialysis patients, even though the revised EBPG consider it necessary to tailor target haemoglobin concentration for individual patients from 11 g/dl to as high as 14 g/dl. The guidelines recommend to individualize anaemia treatment, however, they do not tell how nor do they provide defined criteria. The findings of the third analysis showed that anaemia in a large proportion of dialyzed patients can be effectively managed with a 1x weekly administration of epoetin beta. The 1x weekly dosing regimen appeared to be as effective in maintaining haemoglobin levels as a 2-3x weekly administration. This dosing regimen allows to simplify anaemia treatment, which results in a reduced workload for the medical staff and in a higher convenience for patients.

The guidelines are well implemented in Swiss dialysis centres. However some deviations from the recommendations were observed in respect of the physicians' target haemoglobin levels, epoetin treatment, and iron targets. In contrast to the guidelines, epoetin-naïve patients were predominately treated with a 1x weekly dosing regimen of epoetin beta already at treatment initiation. In two thirds of all patients receiving epoetin beta intravenously, epoetin beta was administered as a 1x weekly regimen, even though there is lack of evidence. A high variability occurred with respect to the iron management. Some physicians tended to observe more carefully the lower limit for serum ferritin levels without restricting upper limits, even though the guidelines recommend an upper limit of 800 µg/l with a target level of 200-500 µg/l. The target range for serum ferritin concentration varied strongly between the different centres and transferrin saturation was not routinely performed in about one third of all participating dialysis centres. A great majority of the dialysis centres did not adhere to the iron targets recommended by the guidelines. It would be advisable to further encourage the implementation of the recommended target iron concentrations in dialysis centres in order to optimize iron management and anaemia treatment in chronic kidney disease patients. Adequate iron management is important for treatment response to ESAs and may result in a considerable dose reduction and cost savings.

The "AIMS" survey proposes some limitations and suggestions for improvement. First of all, several parameters such as dialysis quality (Kt/V), use of ACE inhibitor, CRP (C-reactive protein), and PTH (parathormon) were not assessed. These factors are important contributors to hyporesponsiveness to ESA treatment and they would have been valuable to be assessed as well. Secondly, the survey was not designed to compare the efficacy of the 1x weekly administration to the more frequent administration of epoetin beta. Treatment regimen of epoetin beta, especially dosing interval and route of administration of epoetin beta was allowed to be adapted by the physicians according to the medical needs of each patient. In fact, a separate clinical trial with two randomized treatment groups at study entry would have been necessary in order to compare the efficacy of two treatment regimens, but this would have been contradictory to the main objectives of our survey. Even though these findings have to be interpreted cautiously, they provide valuable information about the relevance and the efficacy of the 1x weekly administration of epoetin beta in Swiss dialysis centres. Finally, there was no control group which may have provided more reliable conclusions in respect of the morbidity and mortality of dialysis patients compared to the healthy population.

A high quality of anaemia control was achieved in dialysis patients in Switzerland with a tendency to normalize haemoglobin levels. Anaemia management in Switzerland adhered to the guidelines, however the implementation of target iron concentration may need to be further improved. Some dialysis centres tailored anaemia treatment according to the clinical profile of each patient as recommended by the revised guidelines, but the great majority aimed at identical target levels for all dialysis patients. The revised guidelines recommend to individualize anaemia treatment, without providing well-defined criterias, though. Tailored anaemia treatment may be rather difficult to be achieved on the basis of individual decisions, efficacy parameters and patients' well-being. Evidence-based target levels for well-defined patient groups have to be established first in order to successfully implement individualized strategies for anaemia treatment in chronic kidney disease patients. However, this will require some more time.

8.4 Conclusions and outlook

The survey "AIMS" represents a simplified tool to perform quality assessments of anaemia management in dialysis patients, which can be easily implemented in each dialysis centre. Furthermore, this tool can be adapted as a computer- or web-based electronic version which facilitates long-term evaluations and quality controls of chronic kidney disease patients. Further algorithms might be integrated with the aim to provide guidance and support in clinical decisions for physicians in order to improve and individualize patient care. The survey may also represent a useful basis in order to establish the Swiss national registry for chronic kidney disease patients. Such tools are essential in order to improve patient care, to facilitate individualized therapy and to provide continuous epidemiological information regarding the development of specific disease areas.

The data of this survey are now used to develop a predictive treatment-response model in dialysis patients, the so-called "artificial neural network model (ANN)". ANNs have been widely used in other domains of clinical medicine in order to solve multidimensional, chaotic problems [164, 165]. Several factors may influence anaemia treatment in dialysis patients. In this model, confounders interfering with anaemia treatment are translated into a complex multidimensional algorithm in order to predict treatment response in dialysis patients. Such a tool can be helpful in everyday clinical practice and may allow a better predictability of treatment changes and medical interactions in dialysis patients. Likewise, it may provide guidance for treatment adaptations on individual basis.

The findings of "AIMS" reveal that a high quality of anaemia control was achieved in the majority of the dialysis patients. However, only one third of all dialysis centres tailored haemoglobin according to the patients' physical condition. The revised guidelines recommend to individualize anaemia treatment, but they do neither explain how, nor do they provide defined specific targets for patient subgroups. Further clinical trials are necessary in order to define specific target levels ensuring the most favourable risk-benefit profile for different patient groups, such as diabetics, patients with cardiovascular disease, young patients and others. A case study showed that different factors might influence the selection of a higher haemoglobin concentration including younger age, gender and physical activity [166]. It would be interesting to further assess in a larger survey whether different haemoglobin concentrations are aimed at for individual patients.

Anaemia is a common risk factor in different diseases. It might be valuable to use the experience made in this survey in other indications. For instance, a survey in transplanted patients would be advisable, since anaemia is insufficiently treated in transplanted patients. Only 10% of all transplanted recipients with anaemia receive anaemia therapy, even though it is of common knowledge that anaemia contributes to cardiovascular risk and impaires patient outcome [36]. The survey should assess anaemia management in clinical practice and further encourage the implementation of the current guidelines in the anaemia treatment of transplanted patiens. Transplanted patients receive high-quality medical care in our country, since they are regularly controlled by nephrologists. However, it would be of importance to better know the clinical practice of anaemia therapy in transplanted patients in Switzerland, since adequate anaemia treatment in these patients may contribute to a better long-term outcome and patients well-being.

It is also known that late referral of predialysis patients to nephrologists often occurs with considerably negative impact on patient survival and other clinical outcomes [8]. An interdisciplinary approach between nephrologists and general practitioners may be favourable in order to improve the early referral pattern and to improve the management of patients during the pre-dialysis period. Anaemia is often underestimated in patients with congestive heart failure as well [167]. The effect of correcting the anaemia was initially assessed in a pilot study, which suggests a benefit from recombinant human erythropoietin (EPO) therapy. However, further investigations are necessary in this field [167]. The prevalence of anaemia in congestive heart failure patients and potential effects of anaemia treatment with epoetin also have to be further investigated in these patients in respect of morbidity and mortality. These investigations could provide further evidence to support the beneficial treatment concept with epoetin in patients with cardio-renal syndrome.

In conclusion, a coordinated approach in the management of chronic kidney disease is required by means of early referral, timely treatment initiation and identification of beneficial target levels in anaemia management, in order to optimize the patient care on an individual basis. Multidisciplinary collaboration and exchange experience of are becoming increasingly important in medicine allowing available resources to be utilized more efficiently. This will positively influence patient outcome and further improve prognosis.

9. Personal remarks

The impetus to write a thesis came from Prof. Hans Kummer during a discussion about ethical aspects concerning a survey which I had developped at that time. He encouraged me to write a thesis based on that specific project. I was delighted with this idea knowing that it would not be easy to realize, since it is unusual to perform a thesis as a sideline. After convincing my superiors at Roche, I kindly asked Prof. Michel Burnier to supervise my thesis. Thereafter, I had to look for a University which would agree to collaborate with an external PhD student. My request was supported by Prof. Marcel Tanner who gave me the possibility to perform my thesis within the interfacultary PhD programme on "Epidemiology" at the Swiss Tropical Institute, an institute associated to the University of Basel.

My PhD thesis was a great experience for me in several points of view. Throughout this work, I could deepen my knowledge about how to design surveys, to prepare research protocols based on the initial objectives, and I learned how to efficiently manage a project. I appreciated the interdisciplinary collaboration with different person, such as nephrologists, statisticians and graphic designers; they all offered me important information for my project and valuable insights into their professional experience.

The interesting and enthusiastic discussions with Prof. Michel Burnier gave me the opportunity to profit from his broad knowledge. This allowed me to further improve my scientific knowledge in the field of anaemia in chronic kidney disease and to better understand the clinical practice in this therapeutical aeria. During the discussions with Prof. Marcel Tanner and Prof. Heiner C. Bucher I learned much about the methodologies of epidemiologic studies. I also got aware of the importance of statistics in epidemiology as well as in medical science, which encouraged me to refresh and deepen my knowledge in statistics. While working on the thesis, I also gained a more critical view in respect of scientific work. I am better able now to judge information independently and to interpret study results better.

These experiences will also have a great influence on my professional life, for I shall be able to provide more valuable advice and suggestions on future medical projects. Likewise, I learned to progress personally in many ways. For instance, I know how to better prioritize, since I performed the thesis concurrently with my regular profession. The experience made in the course of the thesis taught me that it is essential to try out unconventional, new ways and to be a little bit of a visionary. I was also fascinated about the open-minded and human spirit and the broad interdisciplinary knowledge, which I experienced during my work at university. I am convinced that some of this spirit and passion will enrich my personal life.

10. References

1. US Renal Data System. USRDS 1999 annual data reports. National Institute of Diabetes and Digestive and Kidney Disease, Bethesda, MD, 1999.
2. Frei U. and Schober H.J., Bericht über Dialysebehandlungen und Nierentransplantation in Deutschland 1997/1998 [Report on Dialysis Therapy and Renal Transplantation in Germany 1997/1998]. QuaSi-Niere GmbH.
3. Levin A., Thompson C.R., Ethier J., Carlisie E.J.F., Tobe S., Mendelssohn D., Burgess E., Jindal K., Barret B., Singer J., and Djurdjev O., Left ventricular mass index increase in early renal disease: impact of decline in hemoglobin. American Journal of Kidney Diseases, 1999. 34(1): p. 125-134.
4. Besarab A., Bolton K.W., Browne J.K., Egrie J.C., Nissenson A.R., Okamoto D.M., Schwab S.J., and Goodkin D.A., The effects of normal as compared with low hematocrit values in patients with cardiac disease who are receiving hemodialysis and epoetin. The New England Journal of Medicine, 1998. 339(9): p. 584-590.
5. Eckhardt K.-U., Erythropoietin. Oxygen dependent control of erythropoiesis and its failure in renal disease. Nephron, 1994. 67: p. 7-23.
6. Drüeke T.B., Eckhardt K.-U., Frei U., Jacobs C., Kokot F., McMahon L.P., and Schaefer R.M., Does early anemia correction prevent complications of chronic renal failure? Clinical nephrology, 1999. 51(1): p. 1-11.
7. Silverberg D., Blum M., Peer G., and Iaina A., Anemia during the predialysis period: a key to cardiac damage in renal failure. Nephron, 1998. 80: p. 1-5.
8. Valderrábano F., Hörl W.H., Macdougall I.C., Rossert J., Rutkowski B., and Wauters J.-P., Pre-dialysis survey on anaemia management. Nephrology Dialysis Transplantation, 2003. 18: p. 89-100.
9. Mayer G., J. T., Cada E.M., Stummvoll H.K., and Graf H., Working capacity is increased following recombinant human erythropoietin treatment. Kidney International, 1988. 34(4): p. 525-528.
10. Bàràny P., Petterson E., and Konarski-Svensson J.K., Long-term effects on quality of life in haemodialysis patients of correction of anaemia with erythropoietin. Nephrology Dialysis Transplantation, 1993. 8: p. 426-432.
11. Macdougall I.C., Lewis N.P., Saunders M.J., Cochlin D.L., Davies M.E., Hutton D.R., Fox K.A.A., Coles G.A., and D. W.J., Long-term cardiorespiratory effects of amelioration of renal anaemia by erythropoietin. Lancet, 1990. 335: p. 489-494.
12. Locatelli F., Conte F., and Marcelli D., The impact of haematocrit levels and erythropoietin treatment on overall cardiovascular mortality and morbidity - the experience of the Lombarcy Dialysis Registry. Nephrology Dialysis Transplantation, 1998. 13: p. 1642-1644.
13. Foley R.N., Parfrey P.S., Morgan J., Barre P.E., Campbell P., Cartier P., Coyle D., Fine A., Handa P., Kingma I., Lau C.Y., Levin A., Mendelssohn D., Muirhead N., Murphy B., Plante R.K., Posen G., and Wells G.A., Effect of hemoglobin levels in hemodialysis patients with asymptomatic cardiomyopathy. Kidney International, 2000. 58: p. 1325-1335.
14. McMahon L.P., Mason K., Skinner S.L., Burge C.M., Grigg L.E., and Becker G.J., Effects of haemoglobin normalization on quality of life and cardiovascular

parameters in end-stage renal failure. Nephrology Dialysis Transplantation, 2000. 15: p. 1425-1430.
15. NKF-K/DOQI Clinical Practice Guidelines for Anemia of Chronic Kidney Disease: update 2000. American Journal of Kidney Diseases, 2001. 37 (suppl 1): p. 182-238.
16. Harris M.I., Undiagnosed NIDDM: dinical and public health issues. Diabetes Care, 1993. 16(4): p. 642-652.
17. Alberti K.G. and Zimmet P.Z., Definition, diagnosis and classification of diabetes mellitus and its complications. Part I: diagnosis and classification of diabetes mellitus provisional report of a WHO consultation. Diabet Med, 1998. 15(7): p. 539-553.
18. European Diabetes Policy Group. A desktop guide to type 2 diabetes mellitus. Diabet Med, 1999. 16(9): p. 716-730.
19. Morgenson C.E., Christensen C.K., and Vittinghus E., The stages in diabetic renal disease. With emphasis on the stage of incipient diabetic nephropathy. Diabetes, 1983. 32 (suppl 2): p. 64-78.
20. Levy J., Morgan J., and Brown E., Oxford Handbook of dialysis. 2001: Oxford University Press Inc. 4-595.
21. Schönweiss G., Dialysefibel. 2nd ed. 1998, Bad Kissingen: abakiss.
22. Geschäftsbericht Schweizerischer Verband für Gemeinschaftsaufgaben der Krankenversicherer. 2003.
23. Pierratos R., Uldall M., Ouwendyk R., Francoeur R., and Vas S., Two year Experience with the Slow Nocturnal Hemodialysis (SNHD). Journal of the American Society of Nephrology, 1996. 7: p. 1417.
24. Buoncristiani U., Fagugli R., Quintaliani G., and H. K., Rationale for daily dialysis. Home Hemodial Int, 1995. 1: p. 12-18.
25. Schiffl H., Lang S.M., and Fischer R., Dialy hemodialysis and the outcome of acute renal failure. New England Journal of Medicine, 2002. 346(5): p. 305-310.
26. Wetzels A., Colombi A., Dittrich P., Gurland H.J., Kessel M., and Klinkmann H., Hämodialyse, Peritonealdialyse, Membranplasmapherese, ed. 3rd. 1986: Springer-Verlag Berlin Heidelberg New York Tokyo.
27. Blake P.G. and Finkelstein F.O., Why is the proportion of patients doing peritoneal dialysis declining in North America? Peritoneal Dialysis International, 2001. 21: p. 107-114.
28. ERA-EDTA Registry 2002 Annual Report. Academic Medical Center, Amsterdam, The Netherlands. 2004.
29. Report of Dialysed patients in Switzerland. 2002, Schweizerischer Verband für Gemeinschaftsaufgaben der Krankenkassen (Swiss Health Insurers' Association for Shared Tasks: SVK).
30. US Renal Data System. USRDS 2004 annual data reports. National Institute of Diabetes and Digestive and Kidney Disease, Bethesda, MD, 2004.
31. Levin A., Prevalence of cardiovascular damage in early renal disease. Nephrology Dialysis Transplantation, 2001. 16 (Suppl 2): p. 7-11.
32. Portolès J., Torralbo A., and Martin P., Cardiovascular effects of recombinant human erythropoietin in predialysis patients. 1997. 29: p. 541-548.
33. Astor B.C., Muntner P., and Levin A., Association of kidney function with anemia: the Third National Health and Nutrition Examination Survey (1988-1994). Arch Intern Med, 2002. 163: p. 541-548.
34. World Health Organization. Nutritional Anaemias: Report of a WHO Scientific Group. Geneva, Switzerland: World Health Organization, 1968.

35. Lorenz M., Kletzmayr J., Perschl A., Furrer A., W.H. H., and Sunder-Plassmann G., Anemia and iron deficiencies among long-term renal transplant recipients. J Am Soc Nephrol, 2003. 13(3): p. 794-797.
36. Vanrenterghem Y., Ponticelli C., Morales J.M., Abramowicz D., Baboolal K., Eklund B., Kliem V., Legendre C., Morais S.A.L., and Vincenti F., Prevalence and management of anemia in renal transplant recipients: a European survey. Am J Transplant, 2003. 3(7): p. 835-845.
37. Beshara S., Birgegard G., Goch J., Wahlberg J., Wikstrom B., and Danielson B.G., Assessment of erythropoiesis following renal transplantation. Eur J Haematol, 1997. 58(3): p. 167-173.
38. Yorgin P.D., Scanding J.D., Belson A., Sanchez J.A., Alexander S.R., and Andreoni K.A., Late post-transplant anemia in adult renal recipients. An under-recognized problem? Am J Transplant, 2002. 11: p. 313-315.
39. Eschbach J.W., The anemia of chronic renal failure: pathophysiology and the effects of recombinant erythropoietin. Kidney International, 1989. 35: p. 134-148.
40. European best practice guidelines for the management of anaemia in patients with chronic renal failure. Working Party for European Best Practice Guidelines for the Management of Anaemia in Patients with Chronic Renal Failure. Nephrology Dialysis Transplantation, 1999. 14 (suppl 5): p. 1-50.
41. Brenner B.M. and C. R.F., The Production of Erythropoiesis. The kidney, 1991. 2: p. 435.
42. Gregory C.J. and Eaves A.C., Three stages of erythropoietic progenitor cell differentiation distinguished by a number of physical and biologic properties. Blood, 1978. 51: p. 527-537.
43. Muta K. and Krantz S.B., Apoptosis of human erythroid colony-forming cells is decreased by stem cell factor and insulin-like growth factor I as well as erythropoietin. J Cell Physiol, 1993. 156: p. 264-271.
44. Muta K., Krantz S.B., and Bondurant M.C., Distinct roles of erythropoietin, insulin-like growth factor I, and stem cell factor in the development of erythroid progenitor cells. J Clin Invest, 1994. 94: p. 34-43.
45. Rice L. and Alfrey C.P., Neocytolysis contributes to the anemia of renal disease. American Journal of Kidney Diseases, 1999. 33: p. 59-62.
46. Alfrey C.P., Rice L., and Udden M.M., Neocytolysis: physiological down-regulator of red-cell mass. Lancet, 1997. 349: p. 1389-1390.
47. Semenza G.L., Regulation of mammalian O_2 homeostasis by hypoxia-inducible factor 1. Annual Rev Cell Dev Biol, 1999. 15: p. 551-578.
48. Vasquez R. and Villena M., Normal hematological values for healthy persons living at 4000 metres in Bolivia. High Alt Med Biol, 2001. 2: p. 361-367.
49. Kato A., Hishida A., Kumagai H., Furuya R., Nakajima T., and Honda N., Erythropoietin production in patients with chronic renal failure. 1994. 16: p. 645-651.
50. Chandra M., Clemons G.K., and McVicar M., Relation of serum erythropoietin levels to renal excretory function: Evidence for lowered set point for erythropoietin production in chronic renal failure. J Pediatr, 1988. 113: p. 1015-1021.
51. Koch K.M., Patyna D., Shaldon S., and Werner E., Anemia of the regular hemodialysis, patient and its treatment. Nephron, 1974. 12: p. 405-419.
52. Ifudu O., Feldmann J., and Friedman E.A., The intensity of hemodialysis and the response to erythropoietin in patients with end-stage renal disease. New England Journal of Medicine, 1996. 334: p. 420-425.

53. Whitehead V.M., Compty C.H., Posen G.A., and Kaye M., Homeostasis of folic acid in patients undergoing maintenance hemodialysis. New England Journal of Medicine, 1968. 279: p. 970-974.
54. Rao D.S., Shih M.-S., and Mohini R., Effect of serum parathyroid hormone and bone marrow fibrosis on the response to erythropoeint in uremia. New England Journal of Medicine, 1993. 328: p. 171-175.
55. Muirhead N., Hodsman A.B., Hollomby D.J., and Cordy P.E., The role of aluminium and parathyroid hormone in eryhtropoietin resistance in haemodialysis patients. Nephrology Dialysis Transplantation, 1991. 6: p. 342-345.
56. Krantz S.B., Pathogenesis and treatment of anemia of chronic disease. Am J Med Sci, 1994. 307: p. 353-359.
57. Desforges J.F. and Dawson J.P., The anemia of renal failure. Arch Intern Med, 1958. 10: p. 326-332.
58. Hartley L.C.J., Innis M.D., Morgan T.O., and Clunie G.J.A., Splenectomy for anaemia in patients on regular haemodialysis. Lancet, 1971. 2: p. 343-13445.
59. Hocken A.G. and Marwah P.K., Iatrogenic contribution to anaemia of chronic renal failure. Lancet, 1971. 19: p. 95-98.
60. Mann J.F.E., What are the short-term and long-term consequences of anaemia in CRF patients? Nephrology Dialysis Transplantation, 1999. 14 [Suppl 2]: p. 29-36.
61. Foley R.N., Parfrey P.S., and Harnett J.D., Clinical and echocardiographic disease in patients starting end-stage renal disease therapy. Kidney International, 1995. 47: p. 186-192.
62. Foley R.N., Parfrey P.S., Harnett J.D., Kent G.M., Murray D.C., and Barre P.E., The impact of Anemia on Cardiomyopathy, Morbidity, and Mortality in End-Stage Renal Disease. American Journal of Kidney Diseases, 1996. 28(1): p. 53-61.
63. Lin F., Suggs S., Lin C., Brwone J.K., Smalling R., Ergrie J.C., Chen K.K., Fox G.M., Martin F., Stabinsky Z., Bradrawi S.M., Lai P., and Goldwasser E., Cloning and expression of the human erythropoietin gene. Proc Natl Acad Sci USA, 1985. 82: p. 7580.
64. Jacobs K., Shoemaker C., Rudersdorf R., Neill S.D., Kaufmann R.J., Mufson A., Seehra J., Jones S.S., Hewick R., Fritsch E.F., Kawakita M., Shimizu T., and Miake T., Isolation and characterization of genomic and cDNA clones of human erythropoietin. Nature, 1985. 313: p. 806.
65. Sytkowski A.J., Feldmann L., and Zurbuch D.J., Biological activity and structural stability of N-deglycosylated recombinant human erythropoietin. Biochem Biophys Res Commun, 1991. 176: p. 698-704.
66. Dube S., Fisher J.W., and Powell J.S., Glycolisation at specific site of erythropoietin is essential for biosynthesis, secretion, and biological function. J Biol Chem, 1998. 263: p. 17516-17521.
67. Skibeli V., Nissen-Lie G., and Torjesen P., Sugar profiling proves that human serum erythropoietin differs from recombinant human erythropoietin. Blood, 2001. 98 (13): p. 3626-3634.
68. Storring P.L., Tiplady R.J., and Gaines Das R.E., Epoetin alfa and beta differ in their erythropoietin isoform compositions and biological properties. Br J Haematol, 1998. 100: p. 79-89.
69. Halstenson C.E., Macres M., Katz S.A., Schieders J.R., Watanabe M., Sobota J.T., and Abraham P.A., Comparative pharmacokinetics and pharmacodynamics of epoetin alfa and epoetin beta. Clin Pharm Ther, 1991. 50 (6): p. 702-712.

70. Macdougall I., Gray S.J., and Eslston O., Pharmacokinetics of novel erythropoiesis stimulating protein compared with epoetin alfa in dialysis patients. J Am Soc Nephrol, 1999. 10: p. 2392-2395.
71. Summary of Product Characteristics (SmPC) of Darbepoetin alfa. Amgen (Europe) AG, Lucerne, Switzerland.
72. Bommer J., Kugel M., Schoeppe W., Bunkhorst R., Samtleben W., Baramsiepe O., and Scigalla P., Dose-related effects of recombinant human erythropoietin on erythropoiesi: result of a multicentre trial in patients with end-stage renal disease. Contrib Nephrol, 1998. 66: p. 85-93.
73. Besarab A., Reyes C.M., and John H., Meta-Analysis of Subcutaneous Versus Intravenous Epoetin in Maintenance Treatment of Anemia in Hemodialysis Patients. American Journal of Kidney Diseases, 2002. 40(3): p. 439-446.
74. Kaufman J.S., Subcutanous compared with intravenous epoetin in patients receiving hemodialysis. The New England Journal of Medicine, 1998. 339(9): p. 578-583.
75. F. Hoffmann-La Roche Ltd., Product Monograph NeoRecormon. 2000.
76. Besarab A., Flaharty K.K., and Erslev A.J., Clinical pharmacology and economics of recombinant human erythropoietin in end-stage renal disease: the case for subcutaneous administration. J Am Soc Nephrol, 1992. 2(1405-1416).
77. Locatelli F., Baldamus C.A., Villa G., Ganea A., de Francisco A.L.M., and Group o.b.o.t.S., Once-weekly compared with three-times-weekly subcutaneous epoetin beta: results from a randomized, multicenter, therapeutic-equivalence study. American Journal of Kidney Diseases, 2002. 40(1): p. 119-125.
78. Weiss L.G., Clyne N., Fihlho J.D., Frisenette-Fich C., Kurkus J., and Svensson B., The efficacy of once weekly compared with two or three times weekly subcutaneous epoetin beta: Results from a randomized controlled multicentre trial. Nephrology Dialysis Transplantation, 2000. 15: p. 2014-2019.
79. Frifelt J.J., Tvedegaard E., Bruun K., Steffensen G., Cintin C., Breddam M., Dominguez H., and Jorgensen J.D., Efficacy of recombinant human erythropoietin administered subcutaneously to CAPD patients once weekly. Peritoneal Dialysis International, 1996. 16: p. 594-598.
80. Revicki D., Brown R., Feeny D., Henry D., Teehan B., Rudnick M., and Benz R., Health-related qualitiy of life associated with recombinant human erythropoietin therapy for predialysis chronic renal disease patients. American Journal of Kidney Diseases, 1995. 25: p. 548-554.
81. Arzneimittel-Kompendium der Schweiz. 2004.
82. Locatelli F., Aljama P., Bàràny P., Canaud B., Carrera F., Eckhardt K.-U., Hörl W.H., Macdougall I.C., Macleod A., Wiecek A., and Cameron S., Revised European Best Practice Guidelines for the management of anaemia in patients with chronic renal failure. Nephrology Dialysis Transplantation, 2004. 19(Suppl. 2): p. ii1-ii47.
83. Veys N., Dhondt A., and Lameire N., Pain at the injection site of subcutaneously administered erythropoietin: phosphate-buffered epoetin alpha compared to citrate-buffered epoetin alpha and beta. Clin Nephrol, 1998. 49: p. 41-44.
84. Vanregterghem Y., Barany P., and Mann J.F.E., Randomized trial of darbepoetin alfa for treatment of renal anemia at a reduced dose frequency compared with rHuEPO in dialysis patients. Kidney Int, 2002. 62: p. 2167-2175.
85. Macdougall I., Pure red cell aplasia with anti-erythropoietin antibodies occurs more commonly with one formulation of epoetin alfa than another. Curr Med Res Opinion, 2004. 20 (1): p. 83-86.

86. Casadevall N., Nataf J., Viron B., Kilta A., Kiladjian J.J., Martin-Dupont P., Michaud P., Papo T., Ugo V., Teyssandier I., Varet B., and Mayeux P., Pure red cell aplasia and antierythropoietin antibodies in patients treated with recombinant erythropoietin. New England Journal of Medicine, 2002. 346(469-475).
87. Casadevall N., Nataf J., Viron B., Kolta A., Kiladjian J.-J., Martin-Dupont P., Michaud P., Papo T., Ugo V., Teyssandier I., Varet B., and Mayeux P., Pure red-cell aplasia and antierythropoietin antibodies in patients treated with recombinant erythropoietin. New England Journal of Medicine, 1998. 346(7): p. 469-475.
88. Moecks J., Franke W., Ehmer B., Quarder O., and Scigala P., Analysis of safety database for long-term Epoetin-beta treatment:a meta-analysis covering 3697 patients, in Pathogenetic and therapeutic aspects of chronic renal failure, Eds Koch KM S.G., Editor. 1997: NY. p. 163-179.
89. Winearls C.G., Recombinant human erythropoietin: 10 years of clinical experience. Nephrology Dialysis Transplantation, 1998. 13 Suppl. 2: p. 3-8.
90. Albertazzi A., Di Liberato L., Daniele F., Battistel V., and Colombi L., Efficacy and tolerability of recombinant human erythropoietin treatment in pre-dialysis patients: results of a multicenter study. International Journal of Artificial Ogans, 1998. 21(1): p. 12-18.
91. Silberberg J.S., Rahal D.P., Patton D.R., and Sniderman A.D., Role of anemia in the pathogenesis of left ventricular hypertrophy in end-stage renal disease. Am J Cardiol, 1989. 64: p. 222-224.
92. Silberberg J.S., Racine N., Barre P.E., and Sniderman A.D., Regression of left ventricular hypertrophy in dialysis patients following correction of anemia with recombinant human erythropoietin. Can J Cardiol, 1990. 6: p. 1-4.
93. Harnett J.D., Kent G.M., Foley R.N., and Parfrey P.S., Cardiac function and hematocrit level. Am J Kidney Dis, 1995. 26 (suppl 1): p. 3-7.
94. Moecks J., Cardiovascular mortality in haemodialysis patients treated with epoetin beta - a retrospective study. Nephron, 2000. 86: p. 455-462.
95. Moecks J., Franke W., Ehmer B., Quarder O., and Scigala P., Epoetin reduces the mortality? (abstract). Am Soc Nephrol, 1997. 7: p. 222.
96. Ma J.Z., Ebben J., Xia H., and Collins A.J., Hematocrit Level and Associated Mortality in Hemodialysis Patients. Journal of the American Society of Nephrology, 1999. 10: p. 610-619.
97. Xia H., Erben J., Ma J.Z., and Collins A.J., Hematocrit level and associated mortality in hemodialysis patients. Journal of the American Society of Nephrology, 1999. 10: p. 1309-1316.
98. Li S. and Collins A.J., Association of hematocrit value with cardiovascular morbidity and mortality in incident hemodialysis patients. Kidney Int, 2004. 65 (2): p. 626-633.
99. Gouva C.G., Nikolopoulos P., Ioannidis J.P.A., and Siamopoulos K.C., Treating anemia early in renal failure patients slows the decline of renal functin: A randomized controlled trial. Kidney Int, 2004. 66: p. 753-760.
100. Jungers P., Choukroun G., and Oualim Z., Beneficial influence of recombinant human erythropoietin therapy on the rate of progression of chronic renal failure in predialysis patients. Nephrology Dialysis Transplantation, 2001. 16: p. 307-312.
101. Kuriyama S., Tomonari H., and Yoshida H., Reversal of anemia by erythropoietin therapy retards the progression of chronic renal failure, especially in non-diabetic patients. Nephron, 1997. 77: p. 176-185.
102. Eschbach J.W., Cook J.D., Scribner B.H., and Finch C.A., Iron balance in hemodialysis patients. Ann Intern Med, 1977. 87(6): p. 710-713.

103. NKF-DOQI Work group: NFK-DOQI clinical practice guidelines for the treatment of anemia of chronic renal failure. American Journal of Kidney Diseases, 1997. 30: p. 192-240.
104. Drüeke T.B., Barany P., Cazzola M., Eschbach J.W., Grützmacher P., Kaltwasswer J.P., Macdougall I.C., Pippard M.J., Shaldon S., and van Wyck D., Management of iron deficiency in renal anemia: guidelines for the optimal therapeutic approach in erythropoietin-treated patients. Clinical Nephrology, 1997. 48: p. 1-8.
105. Besarab A., Amin N., and Ahsan M., Optimization of epoetin therapy with intravenous iron therapy in hemodialysis patients. Journal of the American Society of Nephrology, 2000. 11: p. 530-538.
106. Danielson B., R-HuEPO hyporesponsiveness--who and why? Nephrology Dialysis Transplantation, 1995. 10 (2): p. 69-73.
107. Caillete A., Barretto S., Gimenez E., Labeeuw M., and Zech P., Is erythropoietin treatment safe and effective in myeloma patients receiving hemodialysis? Clin Nephrol, 1993. 40 (3): p. 176-178.
108. Douglas S.W. and Adamson J.W., The anemia of chronic disorders; studies of marrow regulations and iron metabolism. Blood, 1975. 45: p. 55-65.
109. Albitar S., Genin R., and Fen-Chong M., High dose enalapril impairs the response to erythropoietin treatment in haemodialysis patients. Nephrology Dialysis Transplantation, 1998. 13: p. 1206-1210.
110. Onoyama K., Sanai T., Motomura K., and Fujishima M., Worsening of anemia by angiotensin converting enzyme inhibitors and its prevention by antiestrogenic steroid in chronic hemodialysis patients. J Cardiovasc Pharmacol, 1989. 3 (Suppl.3): p. S27-30.
111. Sanchez J.A., ACE inhibitors do not decrease rHuEPO response in patients with end-stage renal failure (letter). Nephrol Dial Transplant, 1995. 10: p. 1476.
112. Abu-Alfa A.K., Cruz D., Perazella M.A., Mahnensmith R.L., Simon D., and Bia M.J., ACE inhibitors do not induce recombinant human erythropoietin resistance in hemodialysis patients. Am J Kidney Dis, 2000. 35 (6): p. 1076-1082.
113. Schiffl H., Captopril but not losartan interferes with response to erythropoietin in dialysis patients. J Am Soc Nephrol, 1998. 9: p. 330A (abstract).
114. Ikeda Y., Sakemi T., and Ohtsuka Y., Drug-related low responsivness to recombinant human erythropoetin therapy in three patients with end-stage renal disease. Nephrol Dial Transplant, 1997. 12(12): p. 371-372.
115. Besarab A., Bolton K.W., and Brown J.K., The effects of normal as compared with low hematocrit values in patients with cardiac disease who are receiving hemodialysis and epoetin. New England Journal of Medicine, 1998. 339: p. 584-590.
116. Macdougall I., CREATE: new strategies for early anaemia management in renal insufficiency. Nephrol Dial Transplant, 2003. 18 (Suppl 2): p. 13-16.
117. Rao M. and Pereira B.J., Prospective trials on anemia of chronic disease: the Trial to Reduce Cardiovascular Events with Aranesp Therapy (TREAT). Kidney Int, 2003. 87 (Suppl.): p. 12-19.
118. Frankenfield D.L., Johnson C.A., Wish J.B., Rocco M.V., Madore F., and Owen W.F., Anemia management of adult hemodialysis patients in US:result from the 1997 ESRD Core Indicators Project. Kidney Int, 2000. 57: p. 578-589.
119. Valderrábano F., Hörl W.H., Jacobs C., and Macdougall I.C., European Survey on Anaemia Management (ESAM). Nephrology Dialysis Transplantation, 2000. 15 [Suppl. 4]: p. 1-76.

120. Silverberg D.S., Wexler D., and Sheps D., The effect of correction of mild anemia in severe, resistant congestive heart failure using subcutaneous erythropoietin and intravenous iron: a randomized controlled study. J Am Coll Cardiol, 2001. 37: p. 1775-1780.
121. Silverberg D., Iaina A., Wexler D., and Blum M., The pathological consequences of anaemia. Clin Lab Haem, 2001. 23: p. 1-6.
122. Reglement über die Heilmittel im klinischen Versuch. Ergänzende Erläuterungen, in IKS Monatsbericht / Bulletin mensuel OICM. 2000. p. 158-161.
123. Summary of Product Characteristics (SmPC) of Epoetin beta. Roche Ltd. Switzerland.
124. Riffenburgh R.H., Statistics in Medicine. 1999: Academic Press. 3-581.
125. Krankenkassen S.V.d., Epoetin beta Bezüge im Zeitraum von 1.1.2003 bis 31.12.2003. 2004.
126. ERA-EDTA Registry 2001 Annual Report. Academic Medical Center, Amsterdam, The Netherlands. 2003.
127. Erslev A.J., Erythropoietin. New England Journal of Medicine, 1991. 324: p. 1339-1341.
128. Bommer J., Barth H.P., and Zeier M., Efficacy comparison of intravenous and subcutaneous recombinant human erythropoietin administration in hemodialysis patients. Contrib Nephrol, 1991. 88: p. 136-143.
129. Bommer J., Ritz E., Weinrich T., Bommer G., and Ziegler T., Subcutaneous erythropoietin (letter). Lancet, 1988(2): p. 406.
130. The USRDS Dialysis Morbidity and Mortality Study: Wave 2. American Journal of Kidney Diseases, 1997. 30(2, Suppl 1): p. 67-85.
131. Waalen J., Felitti V.J., and Beutler E., Haemoglobin and ferritin concentrations in men and women: cross sectional study. British Medical Journal, 2002. 325: p. 137.
132. Brugnara C., Reticulocyte cellular indices: a new approach in the diagnosis of anemia and monitoring eryhtropoietic function. Cri Rev Clin Lab Sci, 2000. 37: p. 93-130.
133. Macdougall I., Tucker B., Thompson J., Tomson C., Baker L., and Raine A., A randomised controlled study of iron supplementation in patients treated with erythropoietin. Kidney International, 1996. 50: p. 1694-1699.
134. Sepandj F., K. J., West M., and Hirsch D., Economic appraisal of maintenance parenteral iron administration in treatment of anaemia in chronic haemodialysis patients. Nephrology Dialysis Transplantation, 1996. 11: p. 319-322.
135. Fishbane S., Frei G., and Maesaka J., Reduction in recombinant uman erythropoietin doses by the use of chronic intravenous iron supplementation. American Journal of Kidney Diseases, 1995. 26: p. 41-46.
136. Da C.H., Price J.O., Brunner T., and Krantz S.B., Fas ligand is present in human erythroid colony-forming cells and interacts with Fas induced by interferon gamma to produce erythroid cell apoptosis. Blood, 1998. 15: p. 1235-1242.
137. Means R.T. and Krantz S.B., Progress in understanding the pathogenesis of the anemia of chronic disease. Blood, 1992. 80: p. 1639-1647.
138. Meytes D., Gonin E., and Mohini R., Effects of serum parathyroid hormone on erythropoiesis. J Clin INvest, 1981. 67: p. 1263-1269.
139. Lindsay R.M., Burton J.A., and Edward N., Dialyzer blood loss. Clin Nephrol, 1973. 1: p. 29-34.

140. Hoenich N.A., Woffindin C., and Ronco C., Hemodialysers and associated devices in: Replacemetn of renal function by dialysis. Kluwer Academic, Amsterdam: 45h edition 1996, 1996: p. 188-230.
141. Eschbach J.W., Egrie J.C., Downing M.R., Brown J.K., and Adamson J.W., Correction of anemia of end-stage renal disease with recombinant human erythropoietin. New England Journal of Medicine, 1987. 316: p. 73-78.
142. Shinaberger J.H., Miller J.H., and Gardner P.W., Erythropoeitin alert: risks of high hematocrit hemodialysis. ASAIO Trans, 1988. 34: p. 179-184.
143. Raine A., Hypertension, blood viscosity and cardiovascular morbidity in renal failure: implications of erythropoietin therapy. Lancet, 1988. 1: p. 97-99.
144. Furuland H., Linde T., and Danielson B., Physical exercise capacity in patients with end-stage renal disease after normalization of hemoglobin with erythropoietin (EPO). Journal of the American Society of Nephrology, 1998. 9: p. 337A (abstract).
145. Muirhead N., Bargman J., and Burgess E., Evidence-based recommendations for the clinical use of recombinant human erythropoietin. American Journal of Kidney Diseases, 1995. 26: p. 1-24.
146. Locatelli F., Pisoni R., Combe C., Bommer J., Andreucci V., Piera L., Greenwood R., Feldman H., Port F., and Held P., Anaemia in haemodialysis patients of five European countries: association with morbidity and mortality in the Dialysis Outcomes and Practice Patterns Study (DOPPS). Nephrology Dialysis Transplantation, 2004. 19: p. 121-132.
147. Foley R.N., Parfrey P.S., Harnett J.D., Kent G.M., Murray D.C., and Barre P.E., Impact of hypertension on cardiomyopathy, morbidity and mortality in end-stage renal disease. Kidney International, 1996. 49: p. 1379-1385.
148. Parfrey P.S., Foley R.N., Harnett J.D., Kent G.M., Murray D.C., and Barre P.E., Outcome and risk factors for left ventricular disorders in chronic uraemia. Nephrology Dialysis Transplantation, 1996. 11: p. 1277-1285.
149. Moreno F., Sanz-Guajardo D., López-Gómez J.M., Jofre R., and Valderrábano F., Increasing the Hematocrit Has a Beneficial Effect on Quality of Life and Is Safe in Selected Hemodialysis Patients. Journal of the American Society of Nephrology, 2000. 11: p. 335-342.
150. Silverberg D., Wexler D., and Blum M., The effect of correction of anaemia in diabetics and non-diabetics with severe resistant congestive heart failure and chronic renal failure by subcutaneous erythropoietin and intravenous iron. Nephrology Dialysis Transplantation, 2003. 18: p. 141-146.
151. Onkamo P., Vaananen S., Karvonen M., and Tuomlehto J., Worldwide increase in incidence of type I diabetes: the analysis of the data on published incidence trends. Diabetologica, 1999. 42: p. 1395-1403.
152. Amos A.F., McCarty D.-J., and Zimmet P.Z., The rising burden of diabetes and its complications: estimates and projections to the year 2010. Diabet Med, 1997. 14 (Suppl. 5): p. 1-85.
153. Torre-Amione G., Bozkurt B., Deswal A., and Mann D.L., An overview of tumor necrosis factor and the failing human heart. Curent Opinion in Cardiology, 1999. 14: p. 206-210.
154. Donne R.L. and Foley R.N., Anaemia management and cardiomyopathy in renal failure. Nephrology Dialysis Transplantation, 2002. 17 (Suppl. 1): p. 37-40.
155. Ruedin P., Pechère Bertschi A., and Chapuis B., Safety and efficacy of recombinant human erythropoietin treatment of anaemia associated with multiple

myeloma in haemodialysed patients. Nephrology Dialysis Transplantation, 1993. 8: p. 315-318.
156. Caillete A., Barreto S., and Gimenez E., Is erythropoietin treatment safe and effective in myeloma patients receiving hemodialysis? Clin Nephrol, 1993. 40: p. 176-178.
157. Taylor J.K., Mactier R.A., Stewart W.K., and Henderson I.S., Effect of erythropoietin on anaemia in patients with myeloma receiving haemodialysis. Br Med J, 1990. 301: p. 476-477.
158. Mouillet I., Salles G., and Ketterer N., Frequency and significance of anemia in non-Hodgkin's lymphoma patienrs. Ann Oncol, 1998. 9: p. 1109-1115.
159. Oesterborg A., Boogaerts M.A., and Cimino R., Recombinant human erythropoietin in transfusion-dependent anemic patients with multiple myeloma and non-Hodgkin's lymphoma - a randomized multicenter study. Blood, 1996. 87: p. 2675-2682.
160. Beguin Y., Erythropoietin and the anemia of cancer. Acta Clin Belg, 1996. 51: p. 36-52.
161. Pereira B.J., Balance between pro-inflammatory cytokines and their specific inhibitors in patient on dialysis. Nephrology Dialysis Transplantation, 1995. 10: p. 27-32.
162. Goicoechea M., Gomez-Campedera F., and Polo J.R., Secondary hyperparathyroidism as cause of resistance to treatment with erythropoietin: effect of parathyoridectomy. Clin Nephrol, 1996. 45: p. 420-421 (letter).
163. Mandolfo S., Farina M., and Malberti F., Parathyroidectomy (PTX) and eryhtropoietin (rHuEPO) response in anaemic patients with ESRD. Nephrology Dialysis Transplantation, 1997. 12: p. A192.
164. Gabutti L., Burnier M., Mombelli G., and Malé F., Usefulness of artificial neural networks to predict follow-up dietary protein intake in hemodialysis patients. Kidney Int, 2004. 66: p. 399-407.
165. Gabutti L., Vadilonga D., Mombelli G., Burnier M., and Marone C., Artificial neural networks improve the prediction of Kt/V, follow-up dietary intake and hypothesion risk in haemodialysis patients. Nephrol Dial Transplant, 2004. 19: p. 1204-1211.
166. Macdougall I., Individualizing target haemoglobin concentrations-tailoring treamtent for renal anaemia. Nephrol Dial Transplant, 2001. 16 (Suppl. 7): p. 9-14.
167. Silverberg D.S., Wexler D., and Blum M., The use of subcutaneous erythropoietin and intravenous iron for the treatment of the anemia of severe, resistant congestive heart failure improves cardiac and renal function and functional cardiac class, and markedly reduces hospitalizations. J Am Coll Cardiol, 200. 35: p. 1737.

11. List of tables

Table 1-1: Stages of chronic kidney disease classified by glomerular filtration rate 16
Table 1-2: Stages of diabetic nephropathy after Morgenson [19] 17
Table 1-3: Pharmacokinetic parameters of ESAs 27
Table 1-4: Efficacy of the 1x weekly subcutaneous administration of epoetin beta in stable haemodialysis patients 28
Table 1-5: Dosing frequency and route of administration of ESAs 29
Table 1-6: Recommendations of iron targets for anaemia treatment in CKD according to the EBPG 32
Table 3-1: Flow chart of assessments 41
Table 3-2: Structure of dialysis centres in Switzerland and in "AIMS" 44
Table 3-3: Treatment population 47
Table 3-4: Overview of survey interruption 47
Table 3-5: Demographics of the treatment population in "AIMS" 48
Table 3-6: Reported diagnosis of end-stage renal disease in "AIMS" 51
Table 3-7: Reported concomitant diseases in "AIMS"... 52
Table 4-1: Schedule of assessments 57
Table 4-2: Baseline parameters 59
Table 4-3: Route of administration listed by dosing frequency 63
Table 4-4: Efficacy of epoetin beta listed by route of administration (s.c. and i.v.) 64
Table 4-5: Mean serum ferritin levels listed by age for males and females 67
Table 4-6: Distribution of serum ferritin levels 68
Table 4-7: Epoetin dose and haemoglobin listed by serum ferritin level 69
Table 5-1: Overview of targets recommended by the EBPG in anaemia treatment..................... 77
Table 5-2: Schedule of assessments 79
Table 5-3: Diagnosis of end-stage renal disease (ESRD) in "AIMS" 80
Table 5-4: Overview of achieved mean haemoglobin and centre-specific target haemoglobin levels 83
Table 5-5: Distribution of patients according to iron status 85
Table 5-6: Achieved and target serum ferritin and transferrin levels per dialysis centre 86
Table 5-7: Response to epoetin beta treatment in epoetin-naïve and epoetin-pre-treated patients 87
Table 5-8: Resistance to epoetin beta treatment in comparison with responders 90
Table 5-9: Epoetin dose and haemoglobin level in respect of the iron status 91
Table 6-1: Baseline patient characteristics of the 1x weekly and the 2-3x weekly group 100
Table 6-2: Aetiology of end-stage renal disease in the 1x weekly and 2-3x weekly group 101
Table 6-3: Concomitant diseases of the 1x weekly and the 2-3x weekly group 102
Table 6-4: Mean epoetin beta dose and haemoglobin level at baseline and month 1 to 6........... 105
Table 6-5: Mean serum ferritin at baseline and month 1 to 6 105
Table 6-6: Comparison of 1x weekly s.c. versus 2-3x weekly s.c. administration..................... 106
Table 6-7: Comparison of 1x weekly i.v. versus 2-3x weekly i.v. administration 106
Table 7-1: Diagnoses of ESRD in the US, in Europe and in "AIMS" 116
Table 7-2: Prevalence of causes by country 117
Table 7-3: Overview of concomitant diseases in the US and in "AIMS" 118
Table 7-4: Haemoglobin level and mean weekly epoetin beta dose per disease 121
Table 7-5: Overview of achieved mean haemoglobin and centre-specific target haemoglobin levels 122

12. List of figures

Figure 1-1: Regulation of erythropoiesis: Feedback regulation 21
Figure 1-2: Regulation of erythropoiesis as an oxygen-dependent feedback mechanism 22
Figure 1-3: Clinical consequences of anaemia, adapted from Mann [60] 24
Figure 1-4: Molecule of rHuEPO 26
Figure 1-5: Association between haematocrit and risk of hospitalization and mortality in ESRD patients. 30
Figure 1-6: Iron and influence on erythropoietic response 31
Figure 3-1: Proportion of the survey population pre-treated with epoetin beta in relation to all epoetin beta patients per dialysis centre 45
Figure 3-2: Prevalence of diagnosis of ESRD in ERA-EDTA countries compared to "AIMS" ... 45
Figure 3-3: Overview of participating dialysis centres and number of eligible patients 46
Figure 3-4: Distribution of the eligible population by age 48
Figure 3-5: Diagnosis of end-stage renal disease in "AIMS" 49
Figure 3-6: Co-morbidities in "AIMS" at baseline 50
Figure 4-1: Distribution of haemoglobin at baseline and month 6 59
Figure 4-2: Mean haemoglobin levels (± SD) for 6 months 60
Figure 4-3: Mean haemoglobin per decade of age for males and females 61
Figure 4-4: Mean (± SD) and median weekly dosage of epoetin beta for 6 months 62
Figure 4-5: Distribution of mean weekly dosage of epoetin beta per kg (IU/kg) 62
Figure 4-6: Administration frequency of epoetin beta at baseline and after month 6 63
Figure 4-7: Route of administration listed by dosing frequency 64
Figure 4-8: Epoetin beta dosage for subcutaneous and intravenous administration for 6 months 65
Figure 4-9: Haemoglobin levels (± SD) for s.c. and i.v. administration of epoetin beta 66
Figure 4-10: Mean serum ferritin levels (±SD) 66
Figure 4-11: Distribution of serum ferritin at baseline and month 6 67
Figure 4-12: Epoetin dose (±SD) and Hb (±SD) listed by serum ferritin at baseline and month 6 69
Figure 4-13: Inverse relation between epoetin dosage and haemoglobin (±SD) 70
Figure 4-14: Hyporesponsiveness to epoetin treatment at mean weekly epoetin doses of 200 and 300 IU/kg/week 71
Figure 5-1: Distribution of physicians' target Hb and achieved mean Hb level over 6 months 81
Figure 5-2: Distribution of achieved mean Hb and physicians' target Hb 81
Figure 5-3: Proportion of dialysis patients with achieved physicians' target haemoglobin level . 82
Figure 5-4: Distribution of mean serum ferritin levels listed by dialysis treatment 84
Figure 5-5: Distribution of mean transferrin saturation 84
Figure 5-6: Epoetin beta dose and response of epoetin-naïve and epoetin pre-treated patients 88
Figure 5-7: Initial Hb levels in epoetin-naïve patients and after 6 months of epoetin treatment .. 88
Figure 5-8: Change of relationship of Hb and epoetin dose after 6 months in patients with baseline Hb <11 g/dl and epoetin dose <300 IU/kg/week 89
Figure 5-9: Distribution of haemoglobin according to epoetin maintenance dose at baseline 90
Figure 5-10: Epoetin dose by adequacy of iron status 92
Figure 6-1: Mean haemoglobin over time in the two treatment groups 103
Figure 6-2: Mean epoetin beta doses for the 1x weekly and the 2-3 x weekly treatment group . 104
Figure 6-3: Survival curve of dialysis patients for six months 107
Figure 6-4: Patient survival noted at different haemoglobin thresholds 108
Figure 7-1: Cardiovascular diseases of ESRD patients reported in "AIMS" and in USRDS 118
Figure 7-2: Mean haemoglobin by concomitant disease 119

Figure 7-3: Percentage of patients with Hb>11 g/dl and >12 g/dl, respectively, per concomitant disease 120

13. Appendix

List of appendices

Appendix I: Participants of the survey *Anaemla Management in dialysis patients in Switzerland "AIMS"* 147

Appendix II: Questionnaire assessing centre-specific targets for anaemia management............ 148

Appendix I: Participants of the survey *AnaemIa Management in dialysis patients in Switzerland* "AIMS"

Chair and Consultancy:
Prof. Michel Burnier, CHUV, Lausanne
Dr Denes Kiss, Kantonsspital, Liestal
Dr Daniel Teta, CHUV, Lausanne
Prof. Marcel Tanner, Swiss Tropical Instiute, University of Basel, Basel
Prof. Heiner C. Bucher, Clinical Epidemiology, University of Basel, Basel

Particpating Centres:
Prof. Andreas Bock, Dr Kurt Hodel and Dr Stefan Franz, Kantonsspital, Aarau
Dr Susanne Banyai, Hirslanden Klinik, Aarau (now: Kantonsspital, Luzern)
Dr Hans-Rudolf Räz, Kantonsspital, Baden
Dr Claude Descoeudres and Dr Helen Iselin, Salem-Spital, Bern
Dr Hermann Saxenhofer, Lindenhofspital, Bern
Dr Konstantin Vogt, Nephrologie, Bern
Dr Marc Giovannini, Hôpital de la Providence, La Chaux-de-Fonds
Dr Eric Descombes, Hôpital Cantonal, Fribourg
Prof. Pierre-Yves Martin, HCUG, Geneva
Dr Otto Maurer, Regionalspital, Interlaken
Prof. Michel Burnier and Dr. Daniel Teta, CHUV, Lausanne
Dr Beat Von Albertini, Clinique Cécil, Lausanne
Dr Denes Kiss, Kantonsspital, Liestal
Dr Luca Gabutti, Ospedale regionale La Carità, Locarno
Dr Claudia Ferrier-Guerra, Ambulatorio di nefrologia et centro dialisi, Lugano
Dr Andreas Fischer, Kantonsspital, Luzern
Dr Peter Sutter, Hôpital régional, Martigny
Dr Pierre Guibentif, Dr Marc Lévy and Stephane Thomas, Hôpital La Tour SA, Meyrin
Dr Gérard Vogel, Hôpital du Chablais, Monthey
Dr Ewa Cynke, Dialysestation, Münchenstein
Dr Fréderique Barbey and Marie-Thérèse Hudry, Centre d'hémodialyse, Nyon
Dr Hans Freudiger, Centre de dialyse, Onex
Dr Michel Brünisholz, Hôpital Cantonal, Porrentruy
Dr Eduard Blanc, Hôpital Cantonal, Sion
Dr Marcel Schmid, Regionalspital, Visp
Dr Thierry Gauthier, Hôpital Riviera, Vevey
Dr Georges Halabi, Centre Hospitalier, Yverdon-les Bains
Prof. Rudolf Wüthrich, PD Dr Patrice Ambühl, Dr Claude Cao, Dr Marco Miozzari, Universitätspital, Zurich

Project support
Delegates of Roche Pharma (Switzerland) Ltd: Albert-Aubry Cécile, Bruno Surian, Heinz Fivaz, Claude Mounier, Urs Trochsler,
Data management: Michel Pfitzenmaier, Dr Köhler GmbH, Freiburg i.Br.; Dr Stephan Maack, Roche Pharma (Switzerland) Ltd; Nathalie Lötscher, Roche Pharma (Switzerland) Ltd

Project responsibility
Nathalie Lötscher, Roche Pharma (Switzerland) Ltd

Appendix II: Questionnaire assessing centre-specific targets for anaemia management

Fragebogen „Zentrumsspezifische Zielwerte in der Anämiebehandlung"

Faxantwort an N. Lötscher
043 344 05 28

Praxiserfahrungsbericht „Stellenwert der 1x wöchentlichen Verabreichung von Epoetin beta"

Fragenkatalog:

- Ziel-Hämoglobin in Ihrem Zentrum: _____ g/dl

    o Haben Sie unterschiedliche Ziel-Hämoglobinwerte in Abhängigkeit der Begleiterkrankung (z.B. Diabetes, KHK etc.)? Wenn ja, welche?

Begleiterkrankung	Ziel-Hämoglobin (g/dl)
------------------	------------------
------------------	------------------
------------------	------------------
------------------	------------------

- Ziel-Serumferritin in Ihrem Zentrum: _____ ng/ml

    Bemerkungen, Kommentar: _____

- Ziel-Transferrinsättigung in Ihrem Zentrum: _____ %

    Bemerkungen, Kommentar: _____

- Ziel-Blutdruck: _____ / _____ mmHg

Herzlichen Dank für Ihre wertvolle Mitarbeit!

Appendix II - A*naem*I*a* M*anagement in dialysis patients in Switzerland "AIMS"*

Questionnaire "Valeurs cibles dans le traitement de l'anémie rénale"

Veuillez faxer le document rempli à N. Lötscher
043 344 05 28

Rapport d'expérience pratique "Intérêt de l'administration d'époétine beta 1x par semaine dans le traitement de l'anémie"

Questions:

- Valeur cible de l'hémoglobine dans votre centre: _____ g/dl

    o Avez-vous des valeurs cibles de l'hémoglobine différentes en relation des comorbidités (p.ex : diabète etc.)

Maladie concomitante	Valeur cible de l'hémoglobine (g/dl)
-------------------------------	-------------------------------------
-------------------------------	-------------------------------------
-------------------------------	-------------------------------------
-------------------------------	-------------------------------------

- Valeur cible de la ferritine sérique dans votre centre: _____ ng/ml

    Remarques: _____

    _____

- Valeur cible de la saturation de la transferrine
  dans votre centre: _____ %

    Remarques: _____

    _____

- Valeur cible de la pression artérielle: _____ / _____ mmHg

Je vous remercie vivement de votre coopération.

These questionnaires were faxed to the participating centres, accompanied by an introduction letter.

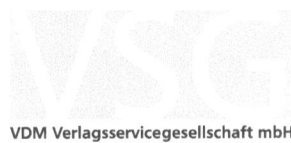

VDM Verlagsservicegesellschaft mbH

Die VDM Verlagsservicegesellschaft sucht für wissenschaftliche Verlage abgeschlossene und herausragende

Dissertationen, Habilitationen, Diplomarbeiten, Master Theses, Magisterarbeiten usw.

für die kostenlose Publikation als Fachbuch.

Sie verfügen über eine Arbeit, die hohen inhaltlichen und formalen Ansprüchen genügt, und haben Interesse an einer honorarvergüteten Publikation?

Dann senden Sie bitte erste Informationen über sich und Ihre Arbeit per Email an *info@vdm-vsg.de*.

Sie erhalten kurzfristig unser Feedback!

VDM Verlagsservicegesellschaft mbH
Dudweiler Landstr. 99   Telefon +49 681 3720 174
D - 66123 Saarbrücken   Fax   +49 681 3720 1749
www.vdm-vsg.de

Die VDM Verlagsservicegesellschaft mbH vertritt

 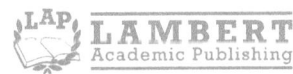 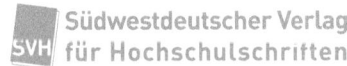

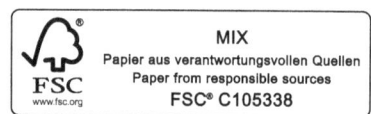

Printed by Books on Demand GmbH, Norderstedt / Germany